PROGNOSIS FOR MISDIAGNOSIS

Eileen Radziunas

DISCLAIMER

To assure the privacy of those described in this true account, while preserving the authenticity of its contents, occasionally facility locations, descriptions, and/or genders have been modified.

TO HUNTER

For making my dream of becoming a grandmother for the very first time come true—and to Connor, Karter, Sawyer, Kiren and Andre for keeping that dream alive. Know that with the arrival of each of you, a special place opened in my heart—one filled with love reserved only for you.

ACKNOWLEDGMENTS

My eyes pool with gratitude toward those family members and friends who demonstrated the wisdom and compassion to recognize, rather than deny, the validity of this illness long before it was accurately diagnosed. With ears that listened so intently they really heard me, well-chosen words which were perceptively delivered when I needed them most and ever-available shoulders to lean on, you gave me the strength I required to endure decades of misdiagnosis. Know that your support and encouragement was immeasurably responsible for my surviving this untreated and indescribably painful challenge that, at times, I was unconvinced was possible—and I love all of you for it.

Inarguably, it was my husband Eddie—my "rock" and best friend—whose influence had the most positive affect of anyone throughout this potentially life-threatening ordeal. More meaningful than the tears one could see that he physically wiped away, were the invisible ones—deep down in my heart—that his endless love and compassion emotionally erased. There are no words to express the dynamic impact he had on getting me through a challenge I'm convinced I never could have survived without him—nor are there those to define the love I have for him for this and countless other reasons.

CONTENTS

INTRODUCTION

"At this very moment, I'm embarrassed to admit I'm a doctor", the physician conducting my moderately invasive procedure shares with unexpected honesty I've been unaccustomed to, during the decades I searched for answers to my medical "mysteries" —but have refreshingly come to realize among the specialists I now see. Having read my chart and reviewed my scans, it is with unconcealed disgust that he adamantly asserts that at least one of my previous practitioners should have been reported.

Somewhat taken off guard by the non-defensive, open-minded attitude he exhibits, my grateful response is, "You, personally, have nothing to be embarrassed about—instead, it is certain members of your profession who owe an apology I will never receive". Placing his arm compassionately on mine, while making direct and purposeful eye contact, he continues, "On behalf of my entire field, I apologize"—and from the pained, tight-lipped look on a face that appears to sheepishly redden by the moment, there is no doubt in my mind that he means it.

What was it in my medical history this doctor found so unconscionable, that just reading it provoked such a strong and assertive stand against the actions of some of his peers—to the point that though personally uninvolved, he felt the need to apologize for them? The answer to this, and far-too-many other questions associated with incorrect diagnoses that patients were resourceful enough to challenge, (and pursue), until their symptoms were accurately identified and appropriately treated, lie within the following pages. They document hard-to-believe, traditionally-held- confidential, true and intimate health accounts patients were brave enough to share—related in ways only individuals who lived them, firsthand, could. Further, they identify the conscientious efforts currently in force by the medical community to aggressively research the causes and potential solutions for medical errors. It is my hope that the combined efforts of all involved will result in a significant reduction of the unacceptably high misdiagnoses statistics repeatedly publicized by the media. Ideally, through accurate diagnoses and appropriate treatment at the earliest stages, patients with rare and difficult-to-diagnose diseases, (including those with atypical presentations), will appreciate the most optimistic prognoses available to current medical science for their specific health challenges.

FOREWORD

As a sixth-grader in the late fifties, I experienced my very first crush—Dr. Ben Casey, star of the then-popular television show. The truth of the matter is that almost every girl my age "loved" him too, evidenced by the popularity of the tunic-like shirts, with buttons in a diagonal line across the top left shoulder, that we all wore. They came in a multitude of colors, many of which had a picture of this kind, gentle, emanating-with-bedside-manner doctor—who could diagnose and cure anything—on the front. As I recall, (which amazes me that I still can!), mine was red and white checked. Stereotypical giddy, pre-teen school girls as we were, we collected Ben Casey posters, pictures, pencils and other reminders of our idol. While the show eventually went off the air and many of those same little girls grew up and found real love, his remarkable and compassionate bedside manner left a lasting impression on the television screens of former viewers' minds, causing them to seek out personal physicians with similar attributes. Though some may argue doing so is idealistic—and that the care he displayed is only reserved for Hollywood—from firsthand experience I disagree. There ARE compassionate and diagnostically proficient Ben Casey clones out there, if you are persistent and selective enough to look for them—a search well worth it in the end. I know mine was!

PROLOGUE

Not All Zebras Live in Zoos: Nightmares of the Misdiagnosed

(A synopsis for those who haven't read my previous books—and a refresher, including updates subsequent to their publications, for those who have).

Living in a body consumed by a serious, misdiagnosed, (or undiagnosed), potentially life-threatening disease—left untreated or inappropriately treated—is a nightmare no one should have to live—yet, in reality, thousands do. Like a prisoner erroneously incarcerated for a crime he did not commit, the undiagnosed or misdiagnosed rare disease patient knows, firsthand, the frustration, shame and trauma of being misjudged. Unlike the unfairly accused, whose sentence is well-publicized, the patient's is far more discreet— a private, internal hell that is his and his alone. If disclosing personal health information and sacrificing pride results in preventing even one patient from living avoidable, (and potentially horrific), consequences of misdiagnosis, I will go to sleep each night with the peace of mind that I have done the right thing. Therefore, directly from the heart of a patient determined to do just that, using words only someone with firsthand experience being grossly misdiagnosed could, I share my true story. And even at that, I fall short—unmistakably aware that despite intensively searching the entire thesaurus of my mind, there are no words powerful and/or descriptive enough to even approach conveying what it was really like, leading me to the conclusion that they just don't exist—in my vocabulary, or anyone else's. Consequently, within the limitations of those available, what follows is an attempt to temporarily transport readers to a world far too many people already know—but one I hope you, personally, never visit firsthand.

* * *

Inescapable and sudden as this kaleidoscope of cascading clear bubbles is, I'm surprisingly not alarmed as it replaces my customary vision—which seems strange given the significant distortion it creates. If anything, I'm both mesmerized and confused as each bubble, in the effervescing waterfall it inexplicably produces, bursts—only to be replaced by a new one.

Rationalizing that I'm probably just tired, I'm slightly taken aback when, glancing over at my husband, (standing just a few feet away), I can't discern his eye color—other than from memory. Before I can verbalize this mystifying observation, he urges me to lie down. With undisguisable concern in his voice, he notes that I don't look well. Though probably overkill, because his persistence is so out of character for someone who has never been an alarmist regarding health issues, I respect his worry—and acquiesce.

As suddenly as they came on, the bubbles cease the moment I enter our bedroom. Deciding to read the newspaper, however, proves to be an exercise in futility. Something's wrong with the print—letters are missing in every word. Unwilling to struggle further by accepting the involuntary challenge and allowing my mind to figure out the omitted letters in these resultant alphabetic blurbs, I give in to unexpectedly sudden, earlier-than-typical fatigue and drift off—but not before the bubbles return again, repeating the same performance.

Birds chirping their sweet, high-pitched conversation outside our bedroom window serve as nature's alarm clock, reminding me that a beautiful new day has dawned—or has it? Enjoyment of this complementary symphony is compromised by my preoccupation with eyes that hurt so badly that if I didn't know better, I would swear they were broiled. Spontaneously reacting to the intolerable pain by lightly massaging my closed lids only intensifies it. Opening my eyes for the first time this morning, my lips become parched, my palms sweat, my heart beats rapidly and my throat dries as I experience a new emotion since first seeing the bubbles— fear.

Knowing that the wall opposite our bed is not blank, it is unnerving that my awareness of the silk flower wreath that hangs in the center of it is from memory only—with no amount of panicky focusing enabling me to visualize it.

Intensifying the distress, my entire body is suddenly invaded by other new and scary symptoms. Inexplicably, I'm no longer able to support my weight on my right leg without falling; voodoo-doll-like pins-and-needles penetrate my body with deep, stabbing head-to-toe pain, my speech is slurred and word retrieval requires over-concentration, usually without success.

I'm urinary incontinent, dizzy, and drool uncontrollably; I experience severe headaches and have difficulty swallowing. There is an unfamiliar deep pain in the back of my neck and I've developed concept dyslexia. During sleep, I'm catapulted off my pillow, involuntarily, by a jolt deep in my head, (accompanied by transformer-blowing-like-sparks). Depth perception distortion, nausea and forceful, uncontrollable limb jerking have also inexplicably begun overnight. Little did I know this was just the start of a diagnostic nightmare that would continue, unresolved, for more than a decade—while testing my determination to live beyond measure.

Initially, I pursued answers from local specialists in numerous fields of expertise. Invariably, when my blood work and scans were normal—which they usually were—it disappoints me to share that, for the most part, I was demeaned and dismissed by the medical community. More gravely ill than I've ever been in my life, I was told I looked too well to be as sick as I claimed and advised to go to lunch with friends to distract myself from focusing on an illness that didn't exist.

One neurologist propped his feet up on his desk and folded his hands arrogantly across his chest, staring silently at me for the first fifteen long, awkward minutes of our initial—(and only!)—visit. Near the conclusion of this virtually speechless consult, I was confused and at a loss as to what had just taken place. Ironically, he found his voice enough to inform me that I did not need the services of a neurologist—nor should I be wasting his time when there were patients who did.

In his report to my internist, he detailed several tests he SUPPOSEDLY conducted—but clearly did not—during the superficial exam he performed in the three minutes I was on the table. Tears stung my eyes, with a few embarrassingly escaping despite my concerted effort to hold them back, as I stumbled clumsily leaving his waiting room, visibly disoriented by the high ceilings and unfamiliar surroundings. But it was the unshed tears, hidden way down deep, that reflected the reality that scared me most—without immediate and appropriate medical intervention, I could die!

In the last paragraph of his report, the neurologist informed my internist that he advised me to see a psychiatrist, in lieu of any clinical findings on his part. Acknowledging that I didn't agree with what he had to say, he documented, "She's a smart woman who will probably reconsider my advice once she gets home, and come around to my way of thinking". (If I weren't too physically ill at the time to find the energy to do so, I think I would have contacted the medical board suggesting that a physician who would silently stare across his desk at a patient—for fifteen minutes—might require seeing a psychiatrist, himself!)

Disgusted, I went elsewhere. Reporting that I was unable to feel the icy temperature of sheets on my lower legs, feet, forearms and hands on a frigid winter night—but could on thighs, trunk and upper arms, a different neurologist told me to "get a grip". According to him, that observation was not indicative of a neurological abnormality—but I had my doubts. Since the bubble incident, our normally cold ceramic tile bathroom floor felt like room temperature against my bare feet. Besides, other doctors noticed instruments were ice cold on some parts of my body and warm on others. Something had changed—dramatically.

Determined to find out what, I scheduled an appointment with a distant neurologist, described to me by another doctor as the "guru of neurology". Unfortunately, I didn't find that to be true. Based on my wide array of symptoms, with surprisingly little objective evidence, he concluded it must be psychosomatic. Though he did get abnormal blood test results on labs he ordered on me, in his opinion they were too few to support organic disease.

A rheumatologist I consulted advised other specialists that I demonstrated no evidence of rheumatologic disease—nor were any future appointments indicated. Another told me to take a vacation on Cape Cod whenever I described my symptoms or the pain associated with them—leaving me feeling dismissed and ignored. One criticized me in his report for showing up with a handwritten list of symptoms. (Ironically, patients are often urged to do just that, today, to avoid omitting important information.)

With each demeaning dismissal, my fear of dying escalated, while my confidence in doctors plummeted. During this uncertain time, I had an especially unnerving experience in which my first conscious awareness, upon awakening at 3:00 A.M., was of my fists clinging to the mattress, clenching it for dear life—fearful of falling off the bed as the room spun around me, leaving me dizzier by the moment. Nauseated as I looked up at a ceiling that appeared to be rotating faster than any carousel I've ever been on, this was quickly becoming a nightmare—but not one I would awaken from any time soon.

With clammy skin, searing bilateral head pain, a racing heart and profuse drooling, there was no doubt I belonged in

The E.R.—but did I really want to go again, for the umpteenth time, as in similar past situations? By now, I knew the routine cold—give some resident the same medical history I've given countless others, expect (and get!), his bewildered expression betraying that he doesn't have a clue, then wait in a stark, curtained-off area while he consults his superior, (which can—and has—taken in excess of three hours in the past). Typically, both doctors return, do blood work and order a scan or two—only to find everything "normal". Sometimes a psychiatrist is recommended due to "non-clinically substantiated complaints". I'm then discharged, every bit as ill as when I arrived, knowing in my heart it will happen again and again—all the while praying I find a physician with the expertise to accurately diagnose, (and effectively treat), whatever is raging inside me—before it is too late.

Looking at my husband sleeping peacefully beside me, I made a decision right then and there. Electing to skip the E.R., I snuggled into the irresistible calm of his lovingly-protective arms.

Being insulted by one-too-many physicians unfamiliar with whatever undiscovered disease I have, has taken its toll. I'm tired of being the target of misplaced frustration generated by an inability to diagnose my "mystery" illness and/or egos that prevent referral elsewhere. While in the past I had little control over their inaccurate assumptions, insensitive treatment and disbelief in my credibility, this is one time I did have a choice—and intended to exercise it. There would be no E.R. for me tonight. What a pathetic and scary commentary on what can happen to a patient repeatedly dismissed—by a profession she did everything in her power to trust—only to encounter consistent rejection.

Desperate, I find myself overcompensating to even approach living the life I once knew—and yet, I have no idea what I'm overcompensating for. There are no words to describe the humiliation and shame I endured by not having a name for this omnipotent force consuming my body. I don't know what caused my world to change so dramatically—nor can I find anyone else to explain it. All I know is a big piece of the "me" I once knew no longer "is'. Replaced by a stranger who has taken up residence in my body, this new occupant is foreign to me—transforming my confidence in previous surroundings into insecurity in a strange new world that requires all my concentration to navigate. Even at that, there are times the intruder—far more powerful than me—appears to be winning.

As determined as I am to understand this bizarre intrusion, more importantly I want it to go away. At the end of every day I pray to wake up to the "old me", with the sense of relief one experiences when they awaken from a nightmare—yet, my nightmare, (or, more accurately, ours'), continued. During twelve of my pre-diagnostic years, my husband was jarred awake at least three times a night, our bed vibrating from my trembling,—but unaware—soundly sleeping body.

With inexplicable continually diminishing eyesight and head pain so intense sleep was impossible, I was desperate for positive distraction to help maintain my sanity. I began journaling during the wee hours—as my household slept. Little did I realize at the time, that these tear-streaked pages would eventually evolve into a book, "But Doctor You're Wrong!"—(but that's jumping ahead).

Meanwhile, my life becomes more challenging by the day—with familiar objects looking different to me than to others. For instance, I asked a doctor's office receptionist if I could borrow her hand sanitizer, as she patiently explained that what I was pointing to was actually the offices' date stamp. Yet, through my distorted vision I could have sworn it looked like the bottle of hand disinfectant my eldest grandson renamed "germ squirt". Situations such as this made me feel like I lived on another planet—among people who spoke a language I didn't understand.

Having exhausted every strategy to convince my physicians of how severely ill I really was, I was running out of options. Out of desperation I obsess with imaginative—though unrealistic scenarios—for attracting their serious attention. For example, one involved those kiosks at malls that allow you to push a button to hear a portion of a CD, prior to deciding if you want to purchase it—only my mind wasn't on music. Instead, I was preoccupied with how diagnostically meaningful it would be, (not to mention affirming to me), if the physicians who didn't believe me—and turned me away untreated—could press a button and experience my symptoms, firsthand, for just a minute. Undoubtedly, they would develop a newfound respect and compassion for ill patients with unidentified and/or misdiagnosed serious conditions.

Guilt interrupts my desperation-induced reverie. I couldn't intentionally impose the beyond-frightening, intensely painful aberrations occurring in body on my worst enemy, even for such a limited amount of time. Although, I must admit I reconsidered that decision at my next consult when, after describing numbness and tingling in my hands, (which I've since learned is neuropathy), the doctor asked me—within earshot of other patients—if I was sure I didn't just have a "deep-rooted masturbation anxiety manifesting in my hands". How does a legitimately ill patient even begin to answer a question like that?

Demonstrating the desperation of a prisoner jailed for a crime he didn't commit, pursuing top lawyers to prove his innocence, I lived the all-too-familiar lifestyle of scared, misdiagnosed rare disease patients everywhere—frantically consulting medical experts nationwide.

Disconcertingly, after multiple plane trips across the United States, (not to mention numerous nights living out of suitcases in expensive, hospital-affiliated hotel rooms), all I had to show for it was a depleted bank account. I was no closer to an accurate answer than when my marathon diagnosis-seeking journey began.

Meanwhile, maintaining my self- esteem became more challenging by the day, as exasperated "professionals" berated me for claiming to be ill—when no tests corroborated it. However, like a mother who knows her own child, and has that extra sense to realize when something is wrong, I know my own body. If some doctor didn't diagnose and treat me soon, my journal may remain unfinished—forever.

What a Difference the Right Doctors Can Make!

A month after an evaluation at one of the most prestigious medical facilities in the country, (where I was again told nothing was physically wrong with me), a new local internist was recommended. Desperate but skeptical, I made an appointment.

Convinced if experienced specialists couldn't figure it out this young physician didn't stand a chance, I soon learned how wrong I was. With the kind of focus a roof collapsing in the next room couldn't penetrate, my new doctor concentrated on every adjectiveI could come up with to describe my symptoms. Unlike other consultations, I did not feel pressured to rush through my medical history—nor cut off, mid-sentence. Indicative of his respect for what patients report, he chose not to rely on past, (often inaccurate and biased), medical records sent from one physician to the next. Clearly this well-credentialed doctor had his own mind and intended to use it—a reassuring approach considering my to–date, undiagnosed status. I was encouraged when he didn't dismiss, as insignificant the shiny, raised, symmetrical, acne-like facial bumps I questioned—because I was sure they were in some way meaningfully connected and, if pursued, could provide a diagnostic clue. However, there was no mistaking his greatest priority: the serious neurological events interrupting my sleep, which he vowed to investigate.

Further, he addressed the severe pain which previous physicians were less vigilant about—in the absence of a diagnosis. Handing me a prescription, I was a little caught off guard—in a good way—by his compassionate and sensitive demeanor. What a refreshing change!

Finally, he assured me that normal blood work would in no way discourage his efforts to pursue an answer to a condition he was convinced had yet to be labeled. He explained that some very serious illnesses don't always show up in the blood, (as I sat there regretting that previous physicians hadn't even considered that). Unmistakably sure that I had a severe form of vasculitis, (an inflammation of the blood vessels—of which there are multiple types), he vowed to get to the bottom of it. And, although I had no reason to believe that, somehow, I did—maybe I just needed to. From that day on, I realized a positive and dramatic change in my medical care. Refreshingly, unlike the others, he did not see me as wasting his time pursuing a condition that didn't exist.

Monitoring me closely, he questioned symptoms no doctor asked me about—and researched them on his own after-hours time. Listening closely and really hearing what I had to say, he methodically pieced the puzzle together, eventually referring me to a neurologist, (because he suspected seizures).

With confirmation of atypical brain wave activity, seizure medication was prescribed—reducing the intensity of the nocturnal arousals and drooling. Further, a cardiologist addressed the abnormal heartbeat, an ophthalmologist discovered optic nerve hemorrhaging and glaucoma, and a gastroenterologist treated vascular intestinal symptoms. Most importantly, a nationally respected rheumatologist diagnosed Behcet's disease, (a severe form of vasculitis that can lead to blindness, seizures and strokes—among other serious symptoms). It is one of over 7,000 rare diseases currently recognized by The National Organization of Rare Disorders, (NORD). Further helping to confirm this diagnosis, this latest work-up I tested positive for the genetic marker HLA-B51, (a blood test often indicative of Behcet's—one no other rheumatologist had ordered).

I was prescribed chemotherapy and steroids at my first visit, approximately a decade ago—and have remained on some of those potent drugs ever since. Anti-inflammatory infusions have also subsequently been introduced. (Ironically, in the past both neurologists and rheumatologists told me never to come back—yet their specialties are commonly known to diagnose Behcet's).

I will never forget the day I first saw this rheumatologist. In disbelief, my husband and I listened, spellbound, as he explained, definitively, what I had and, more importantly, how to treat it— which is all I ever asked for from the beginning of this diagnostic nightmare.

Fast Forward Two Years

I'm somewhat awed, but not in the least bit insecure, as Eddie and I are asked to join a semicircle of interventional neuro-radiologists at a well-respected out-of-state medical institution. The purpose of this visit is to review brain scans conducted over the years, in the hope of solving my still undiagnosed neurological medical mystery. My confidence in attending this forum is that while they know—and can technically explain what they see on the scans—I know my own body and can detail what I experience, daily, better than anyone else—so bring it on, I'm ready!

Methodically, for well over an hour, the head specialist scrutinizes every image, shocking us with a revelation we are not expecting—but one that unmasks a world of mystery associated with my case. In an awed, "Aha" voice, he verbalizes that the "bubble" incident was actually a deep, undetected brainstem stroke—accounting for every symptom I described—to over 100 physicians—for more than a decade. As he places a comforting hand on my arm, my glistening eyes look into his, appreciatively—while everyone in the room is momentarily stunned silent, trying to absorb the magnitude of what was just revealed. Once they do, it feels like the entire staff is giving me an emotional group hug. Reflected in the too-impossible-to-believe looks in their eyes is the realization of what I'd endured independent of necessary medical intervention and supportive stroke rehabilitation—while having done everything I could to obtain it.

A proverb associated with medical schools since the 1950's is: "When you hear hoofbeats, think horses, not zebras". The premise behind it, in relation to physicians, is that when diagnosing a patient, they should first consider the most expected probability rather than the unusual. While to some this thinking is inarguably valuable, consulting a physician who strictly adheres to that mentality—rather than recognizing there are times someone is so ill that they must cut to the chase and consider the rare possibilities immediately—can be a death sentence for a "mystery illness" patient who requires outside-the-box thinking from the moment they walk into the doctor's office.

As you proceed to read this book, please do so knowing every minute of time and ounce of courage it took to share this true account is dedicated to currently undiagnosed and/or misdiagnosed patients—with my prayers that their accurate diagnoses are imminent so that they never have a story like mine, (or those of the other patient's accounts included), to tell.

CHAPTER ONE

I'm Out of Here!

"Knowing what must be done does away with fear." — Rosa Parks

Age appropriately consumed by the literal thinking of a child, there was a time when the phrase, "I could have kissed the ground I walked on", repulsed me. But I'm no longer a child—and my thoughts have matured to those of an adult. Unlike so many years ago, (a time it is surprising I can still recall in such detail), my brain cells are far less impressionable—no longer resurrecting disgusting visuals I'd rather not entertain—like kissing a filthy, germy sidewalk. Age has taught me otherwise. As a result, I allow my thoughts to think those very words that once repulsed me, as my there-is-no-escaping-this-hospital-without-permission-wristbands are snipped off and I'm discharged from a nationally acclaimed, though unfortunately not particularly nearby medical institution. As they are, a feeling of exhilaration infiltrates my veins with rivers of relief that I can't see—but sense from head-to-toe. Inarguably, most patients are understandably grateful to go home after a hospital stay, particularly such a long one, but my exuberance is disproportionate to what I'd consider within normal ranges for this situation. With an ear-to-ear smile and incessant excited babbling, one would think I was just released from prison!

Let me back up. Though I'd been warned prior to my eight-day stay that EEG, (electroencephalogram), video monitoring would involve some restrictions, I didn't realize I was going into solitary confinement! After arriving at the hospital and checking in at the Admission's Office, I'm escorted to what will be my home away from home for the next week-plus. Located at the end of a long, grey-walled corridor decorated with subtle, soothing artwork, it is intentionally situated far from the nurses' station to provide a quiet environment conducive to sleep, which is an essential element of this study.

The private quarters come equipped with a bathroom, nightstand and a metal locker labeled with my name written on a fresh piece of irregularly-bordered, torn but clean masking tape as opposed to the yellowed remnants of those of previous patients whose names have been torn off—leaving pieces of curled tape not completely removed, over which mine is superimposed, reminding me that I'm not the first patient to use it. Optimistic from this visible indication that others completed the same study and got to go home, I focus on this positive thought as I place my clothes in the locker.

Just as I locate space for my last item on the top shelf, a nurse enters the room to review my current medication list, verify past surgeries, inquire as to whether I have a Living Will and query if I've had a flu and/or pneumonia shot. She then documents the date of my last PAP smear, which is current. (Excuse me, but I thought I was admitted for brain wave testing, not to provide a course in ANATOMY 101 for medical students!).

As I'm asked to sign the form she just completed, after scrutinizing it to ascertain that she accurately interpreted and transposed the information I provided, a gentleman appears at the door to take me down the hall to a tiny room where EEG leads are glued to patients' scalps. An hour, (and no pain, later), he returns me to my room, looking like a combination of an alien and someone about to be electrocuted. Even with the white mesh cap he provided, it is impossible to miss the numerous multi-colored, vermicelli-like thin wires underneath—which I've already managed to get tangled in. Though I haven't counted them, I would guesstimate there are in excess of twenty in my unattractive, but all-important headdress. If wearing this contraption means that my doctor can shed some light on what is forcefully jerking me awake, multiple times a night and, more specifically, treat it, it will be well worth the hospitalization.

This thinking quickly changes when I'm informed that I can't get out of bed during my entire stay. Excuse me, do they realize we're talking at least seven days? Have they heard of muscle atrophy? What about showers and bathroom needs? Fortunately, my physician arrives just as some very uncomfortable scenarios start to clutter my mind in an inarguably negative way. After MUCH pleading, I convince her, reluctant as she is to agree, that I don't need to be on bed restriction, given that my "events", (as everyone on the floor refers to them), only occur in my sleep. Compromising, I am given bathroom privileges as long as I don't let the other patients know, since many are dealing with daytime episodes which the cameras could miss if they were in the restroom when they occurred. That works for me! Besides, the way I see it, I've already had to agree to a huge concession—no showers for the entire duration of my stay because the wires can't get wet. (I can almost feel my hair itch, at the mere thought of going seven or more days without washing it!) At the very least, I suppose I should be grateful for sponge baths.

From my perspective, the first few days of hospitalization are uneventful. According to my physician, however, there are some irregularities registering on my electroencephalogram, (which I don't physically detect), related to slowing of the brainwaves. Because distinct seizure activity is not recorded, she decides to discontinue the seizure medications—with the intent of trying to initiate an event.

Initially, I notice no changes subsequent to the medication withdrawal. But gradually, over the next two days, unmistakably abnormal symptoms begin to surface. My limbs forcefully jerk, I drool profusely in my sleep and the buzzing chills I typically experience throughout my body increase in intensity. However, it is the visual changes I detect by the third day of withdrawal from my medications that scare me most.

Trying to focus on the calendar hanging on the wall facing the foot of my bed, the one I've been relying on as I count the days until discharge, I struggle to make out the numbers, which, frighteningly, I can no longer do. Denial supersedes logic as I convince myself that I am probably just tired, but denial is only effective to a point.

When my breakfast arrives, I can feel my face flush with the heat of embarrassment, cognizant of being on camera, (the one videotaping the EEG), as my fork misses its target, repeatedly. Like an uncoordinated toddler learning to negotiate utensils for the first time, I'm equally unsuccessful. As every stab of the fork clinks awkwardly against the plate, missing the pieces of French Toast it aims for by about an inch, it soon becomes abundantly clear that I'm not seeing things where they are—instead, about a half inch to an inch off. Frustration and embarrassment become overridden by escalating fear that replaces both emotions. Clumsily grasping the dome-shaped inverted lid, the one with thermal characteristics intended to keep food warm during transport, (but usually doesn't), I place it over my uneaten food, askew that it may be, in disgust.

Trying to distract myself from a potential reality too serious to face, permanent compromised sight, I reach for the crossword puzzle I started last night. Could I have chosen a more illogical activity at the moment? The clue letters are beyond deciphering—seemingly melting into each other as unrecognizable blurbs of print. Tossing the book in frustration onto my side table—with as many unsolved, blank squares as when I first reached for it—I welcome the timely appearance of my physician at the foot of my bed.

My voice trembling uncontrollably, I blurt out, "I'm losing my vision! Please put me back on the seizure drugs." Though sympathetic about my serious observation, she explains that by withholding those medications just a few more days, the chances of capturing an event will increase. Assuring me she will then resume the most effective prescription regiment indicated for the type of seizures I am experiencing, she exits just as a student social worker enters the room to discuss my rapidly deteriorating sight.

Our conversation is long and surprisingly relaxing, given the gravity of the topic. At one point, I volunteer that if I lose my sight completely, I will probably rely heavily—during the initial adjustment stages—on her specialty. Nodding her head up and down while compassionate, knowing eyes meet mine, demonstrates her non-verbal, but accurately interpreted agreement. Exiting the room after thanking me for all I taught her about Behcet's Disease, I silently pray I never need the services of her profession for sight loss, a condition I implore God never to let come to fruition.

Meanwhile, the longer my hospital stay continues, my impatience with the restrictions intensifies. With every freshly showered medical professional who enters my room, from whom the pleasant aroma of soap still lingering on their skin emanates in an impossible-to-miss, squeaky clean scent as they approach me to take vitals—I want to snap, "How would you feel if you hadn't washed your hair in eight days?" As it is, I'm here longer than originally promised because I haven't had a major event register on the monitors yet, though they do see abnormalities. The spontaneity of the episodes is problematic in that none of us can predict when they will occur. I can go for two weeks without one and then have eight in one night. Cognizant of this, but still determined to capture one, my physician, (whom undoubtedly has only my best interests in mind), insists that I stay a few extra days. Respecting her genuine concern, I agree reluctantly, knowing the priority is an accurate diagnosis.

Disappointingly, doing so means giving up the first few days of our annual Cape Cod vacation, a tradition our family has enjoyed for decades. Anticipation of the scent of the unmistakable beachy air, combined with the squawking of seagulls, foghorns in the distance, gritty sand between our toes, salty lips, long walks on hard packed, firmer sand where the ocean kisses the shore and re-acquainting with friends we've known for decades, (having purchased the same timeshare weeks), are the only things that keep me going through this restrictive in-patient EEG admission—but enough is enough, I want out!

Certainly, not making my stay more tolerable, unlike other hospitalizations I find the nursing staff, (or at least those assigned to me), egotistical and unfriendly—not to mention uncompassionate. My guess is that because they are employed by a facility with such an impressive and well-known reputation, some of them feel entitled—unfortunately misusing power in a way that effects patients adversely. For example, when I ask for a basin of water to wash up, I'm confronted with, "Why? It's not as though you have a job to get to."

While acute hearing is an undeniable blessing I never take for granted, there are times I'm not meant to hear things that I regrettably do. Last night I overheard a staff member in the hallway telling another that she no longer has any intention of bringing me towels when I request them—and that I will just have to wait until she decides it is time to get washed up.

Sticking to hot, sweaty sheets in the hot hospital bed the next morning, I politely ask to get cleaned up. With a smirk on her face that I find annoying, she regurgitates word-for-word, the same response I overheard her tell the staff member in the hall the day before. Suddenly overwhelmed as I consider that I'm attached with glue to electrodes I can't remove, while my personal hygiene is controlled by "professionals" who show no regard or compassion for what it is like to be in my place, the powerlessness of my position causes my eyes to swell with unspilled, but nevertheless present, tears.

I can't wait to get out of here, a feeling that only exacerbates as I hear her describe, (actually it sounds more like gloating), to her peer—once again in the hallway, but within earshot—how she handled my request for towels today. Adding insult to injury, she concludes with a comment about finding it inconvenient that I wanted to use the bathroom. "If she asks too frequently, we'll catheterize her. See how she likes that!", one laughingly threatened as she walked down the hall. Having heard her, I drastically reduce my fluid intake, (so as not to fulfill her sarcastic promise), yet all the while knowing I'm risking the unlikely possibility of dehydration. I say unlikely because my physician has initiated discharge procedures to take effect within the next twenty-four hours.

A day later I'm wheeled out the semi-circle main entrance of the hospital. Too weak from immobilization to run, once I'm allowed to stand I have to make a concerted effort not to kiss the ground, fearful that displaying such honest emotion would lead to re-admission for further evaluation. This was the worst hospitalization I've ever had the misfortune of encountering; patients shouldn't feel like prisoners, which I unmistakably did. Far more staff training to promote awareness and compassion for patients undergoing tests requiring tethering is indicated. While my physicians were very compassionate and understanding, others in charge of direct patient care, on the wing I was assigned to, desperately need a tutorial—perhaps a few days in a clinical admission undergoing the same restrictive environment. There is a lot to be said for firsthand exposure.

Going directly from the hospital to Cape Cod, in our previously packed car, I crave and drink lemonade—stopping multiple times, undoubtedly on the brink of dehydration, if not already there. Unfortunately, my medical concerns are far more serious than a temporary lack of fluids, which I successfully replenish. Looking at the radio station numbers on the car's front panel, (or, more accurately, where I know them to be), my skin ripples with panic- induced goosebumps at the realization that even in such close proximity, I can't read them. Undeniably, my sight has diminished considerably since admission. Please God, don't let it get any worse!

Arriving at the beginning of the Cape, my adult "Magical Memory-Making World for the Summer", oddly the landmarks I've come to recognize over the decades—as exciting reminders that we are almost at our condo—no longer exist, at least not within my focus. Like a child whose recollection unmistakably realizes we are near his favorite candy store, despite not having been there in an entire year, I stare relentlessly out the car window willing my mind to find the familiar, which it does not—at least not with my current vision. Acutely aware of my too-frightening-to-consider potential reality, Eddie begins to read aloud the names of the little flower cottages, lined in a row, that we traditionally do as a family—knowing seeing them is an exciting sign that we are only five minutes from our destination. Actually, it was our daughter Storey who started reciting each one when she was a little girl— and I guess that secret desire of parents, that little part that many of us have but won't admit to—the one that wants to keep their children young forever—is the reason we continue the tradition. Though now grown into a successful young woman, the memory of a time that seems like only yesterday, but really wasn't, transforms our faces into smiles and admittedly has been known to cause our eyes to fill with happy tears, from the recollection of a special time in our lives—one that we will never forget, nor would we want to.

Frighteningly, it just isn't the same this year with my vision incredulously deteriorating right before my inexplicably compromised eyes. There is no disguising the understandable panic it induces. Though the denial that automatically kicked in at the hospital might have been temporarily semi-effective, one can only stretch denial so far. Unable to read any road signs, no matter how I try, I can't avoid the honest but unnerving question that only the privacy of my mind has dared to consider so far: How can I ever get behind the wheel of a car again if my eyesight remains as compromised as it is at the moment?

Arriving at our condo unit at the same time as Storey and her boyfriend Ravi, tears that welled for far-too-many hours—exerting pressure like water in a drooping, over-filled water balloon about to burst—can no longer remain unshed behind my bulging, uncomfortable eyelids. As Storey hugs me, I unsuccessfully struggle to make out her features, (which, at this point I can only appreciate from memory), before the floodgates involuntarily let loose.

Seated at one of our favorite restaurants later that day, my concern and frustration escalates as Eddie has to read the menu to me, making what is intended to be an enjoyable experience a negative reminder of the threatening reality I'm not ready to verbalize, but may have no choice but to face.

Desperate to take some control over a situation that I feel I have none, I do something extremely out of character for my, at times, annoyingly anal rule-follower personality. Defying the discharging neurologist's orders to remain off seizure drugs, due to lack of a captured "event" while hospitalized, I decide to resume them.

Ingesting the medications, it is with little optimism considering I have no medical background. Instead, I'm a desperate patient going out on a potentially hopeless limb, willing my body to respond positively. From my perspective, what do I have to lose? As my first patient-prescribed dose works its way down my Sahara-Desert-dry-from-nervousness esophagus, I silently say a prayer, leaving my fate in the God I trust.

A few days later while seated at a wooden table in another family–favorite restaurant, (which judging by the unevenly carved, multiple personalized initials—taking the place of a tablecloth on the surface of the well-distressed wood—were not a part of the original design), I'm suddenly nostalgic, reminiscing that our children probably sat at this very table, years ago, in booster seats. Distracted as I am by my "mom memory brain cells" the familiarity of this restaurant activates, it takes a moment to notice the puzzled, inquisitive looks exchanged by my family which, when I do, transport me from whatever far-away planet I was temporarily, (and solely), visiting, back to reality—and then I realize the reason for the confusion registered on each of their faces, (which, surprisingly, my eyesight is able to detect). I just ordered for myself off the same size print, glossy menu that I couldn't read only two days earlier! No longer undecipherable blurbs, with about as much meaning as if I were trying to order in a foreign country whose native language I am unfamiliar with and where no English is spoken, the words are clearly within my visual reach. Though almost afraid to believe it myself, I can't—nor don't want to—stifle the small glimmer of hope illuminating my heart from deep within, a glowing, healing light I can't see but feel inarguably. Unable to prevent myself from entertaining the remote possibility that the seizure medication is responsible, I sleep better tonight than I have in a week.

The next morning, (with my continued self-treatment), there is no denying improvement in my vision, as optimism replaces fear I've never before experienced. While I'm not describing visual restoration to where it was prior to the bubble incident, (brainstem stroke), at least I can now see to the degree I could before my seizure medications were discontinued at the hospital—blurry, but able to read—and I'll take that! Needless to say, the sight improvement made my vacation.

Chapter TWO

Forever in My Heart

"Never underestimate the pain of a person, because in all honesty, everyone is struggling. Some people are better at hiding it than others." —Will Smith

"In the end, it is not the years in your life that count. It is the life in your years." —Abraham Lincoln

As Stacey and Tim stand beside me waiting while I unwrap the large colorfully-decorated box, the looks on their faces remind me of little children—bursting inside, impatiently watching their parents open a secret gift they made for them at school and kept hidden under their beds until the holidays. Demonstrating the same antsy I-almost-have-to-sit-on-my-hands-and-tape-my-mouth-shut-behavior, to avoid blurting out the surprise prematurely, I have no guesses as to what it is—but the unmistakable feeling of their focused eyes watching my every move tells me they anticipate quite a reaction. Reaching in the eventually-unwrapped box, tears stream down my cheeks when I read the words "Baby's First Christmas" on a pewter picture frame ornament. Like electricity unexpectedly turned back on after a storm, I suddenly see the light when the realization that I'm about to become a grandmother, registers. Hugging them, I look over at Eddie and immediately know from the expression on his face—the one experienced spouses can't hide from each other—that this is not news to him. Apparently when he accepted the St. Nicholas role at a family reunion Christmas party several weeks ago, Stacey whispered in his ear that she had a present for "Santa"—and swore him to secrecy. Too excited to be annoyed that this news I'd been praying for was kept a secret from me until now, I'm touched by the extremes they went to in their successful attempt to make it the unexpected and beyond-words surprise that it is. A grandmother—does it get any better than that, I ask myself rhetorically, as I continue unwrapping child safety devices for electrical outlets and kitchen cabinets, children's story books and various other grandmother essentials. Unable to concentrate on anything other than the recurring thought that my "baby" is having a baby, I feel euphorically blessed beyond words as I lie in bed that night praying it isn't a dream—and that when I wake up in the morning, this grandmother-to-be will have some shopping to do!

Several Months Later

Instantaneous love flushes through my veins the minute I first lay eyes on our grandson. Convinced there couldn't be a sweeter, more cherubic little face on the entire planet, my eyes fill with relieved tears upon learning he and our daughter are both fine. Little do I know that the prayer I say, at this unforgettable moment, will be repeated five more times—with the arrival of each additional grandchild. Words can't do justice to what it means to be a grandmother—how fortunate I am to live the feeling, firsthand. Yet, the unpredictability of life throws us disconcerting curves when we expect them least. The call I come home to on my message machine sends hair-prickling chills down my spine, like chalk screeching against a chalkboard. It is from my cousin, reluctantly informing me my dad was rushed to the hospital this morning—by ambulance—after discovered on the floor of his senior living apartment, located in the same building as her mom's. "No, not my dad", my inner voice insists—the one that responds with the denial and magical thinking of a child who blocks her ears to avoid the truth, silently pretending what she heard is happening to someone else—not HER dad.

Words don't exist to adequately describe the depth of my relationship with my father. He is my friend, confidant and, in addition to Eddie, the main man in my life. We store memories in our hearts that are exclusively ours. As his only daughter, and the eldest of six children, we were inseparable during my childhood. When I got married, we maintained that relationship by visiting regularly. He comes to our home for "sleep-overs", takes me to breakfast once a week, travels with us, enjoys Eddie and the girls, and so forth.

One of the most difficult thoughts for me to ever process—one that I do everything I can to distract myself from even materializing in the deepest, most sensitive and private chambers of my mind—is the reality that the day will come when he is no longer here—and my heart cries, prematurely, realizing I will never be ready for it.

Just as I hang up the phone from listening to my cousin's message—before I even have the opportunity to fully digest what she said—it rings. Some physician whose name doesn't even register as familiar to me is on the other end. Apparently, he is calling from the hospital my dad was taken to—inquiring as to when I saw him last. Sharing that it was two days ago, he goes on to say that, based on how recent it was, I must already be aware of how very ill he is. "Shut up!", my head silently screams. I don't want to hear what he is saying because I know he is right. My dad, who adamantly refuses to see doctors due to a bad experience in the past, has been growing weaker and paler by the day. I've heard his labored breathing over the phone, probably because it was easier for me to detect without visual, in-person distractions. He no longer participates in his normal activities and his once hearty appetite is almost non-existent. Notoriously independent, he now welcomes my brother Jim, Eddie and I doing his laundry and errands. On the way home from work Eddie picks up clothes he needs washed and returns them clean the next day. With grateful appreciation, he repeatedly thanks us for making "this" easier for him. Suddenly "this" takes on new meaning. It is a word we all know his connotation of but our lips are unable to bring themselves to utter. Dad and I have had more private, never-to-be-shared talks from the heart lately, than ever. He knows his time is running out. All the signs are there, including some he chooses not to share at the moment. Consequently, though scared I'm not in the least bit surprised to hear the doctor on the phone—telling me we will talk when I get to the hospital.

With my adrenalin spiking, it takes monumental restraint to resist the urge to get behind the wheel of the car and make a beeline to the hospital. Instead, I miraculously exercise the presence of mind to call Eddie. Coming straight home, he picks me up, with our only stop getting my brother Jim on the way.

Walking through the lobby adjacent to a cheery gift shop, with Mylar balloons floating erratically across the ceiling with every move shoppers make, my gut tells me we won't be buying one on the way out. Unlike other purchasers, I'm not predicting a reason to celebrate.

With sweaty palms and a virtually saliva-free dry throat, I identify myself to the charge nurse in I.C.U. who immediately summons the physician who called me. As he ushers us into a small, private room and shuts the door, there is one thought and one thought only occupying my mind—this CAN'T be a good sign! The impossible-to-disguise expression on this man I've never laid eyes on before says far more than my ears are prepared to hear. But, at the moment, avoidance is not an option—the time to face reality is here, despite the fact that I'm not ready for it—nor will I ever be. As gently and compassionately as possible, all the while his eyes pooling, he explains what we already know but don't want to accept. Our dad is morbidly ill, with only hours, at most, to live. Informing us that he has had a massive stroke, the doctor does his best to prepare us—not that anything he says adequately could—for what to expect when we see him. He is not conscious and as a result, will not know we're there. To me, he looks like he is sleeping—yet attached to more monitors than I'm sure he's ever seen—let alone would agree to. Sitting next to him, I take his hand and never let go until he passes a few hours later. Numb from head to toe, I leave the hospital knowing the open wound in my heart resulting from this loss, will leave not only a permanent scar—but memories only two people share—and I intend to keep it that way.

My world as I knew it just turned upside down. How can life ever be the same without him? Please God, help me through this.

Convinced that nothing could make me smile as I face one of the most devastating–beyond-words-challenges-of-my-life, my only grandchild—now just over a year old—proves otherwise. The minute Stacey and Tim walk in, somehow holding him in my arms miraculously does. Gazing into the adorable face of the little boy who has come to mean more to me than life itself, his innocent eyes and mine meet each other—and sadness is in competition with an overwhelming love that somehow soothes me—in a way his tender age could never comprehend, nor my adult one thought possible. With a look of appreciation in Stacey and Tim's direction, as I cuddle my him close to me, I verbally share what my mind believed to this point—but never expressed to them—that I'd thought my lips were physically and emotionally incapable of contorting into a smile—but that incredulously seeing him made it happen. Stacey's compassionate and knowing response is, "We were counting on that".

Further comforting, Storey and Ravi arrive within the hour. We are especially touched that despite having to travel the next morning to an important out-of-state work assignment—and that he had just met my dad a few weeks ago—Ravi still came to the wake the night before the funeral. His compassion and sensitivity toward Storey and the rest of our family warms my heart—particularly now. For Storey's sake and that of all of us, I'm so grateful he got to meet "Pa-Pa Red" in person before dad's passing—(and especially that he and Storey met!).

At his service, my brother Al considerately asks me to stand next to him as he gives the eulogy—but I can't. My legs are gelatinous, wobbly and ready to collapse at any moment, as my involuntarily trembling body reflects the lack of control I'm experiencing. Though only vaguely aware, in this surreal setting, of the hand one of my sisters-in-law compassionately extends and places in mine, the way I relentlessly cling to it demonstrates how much it is appreciated—even if on a subconscious level—as I listen to Al's words so lovingly describe our dad. When he gets to the part about wanting to be just like him, our moist eyes meet with firsthand, knowing understanding.

Though the words he chooses come from his lips, he is speaking straight from his heart. I'm proud of him for articulating, at this difficult time, sentiments I also own—but my shaking, in-shock body refuses to allow me to verbalize. How grateful I am for the beautiful and well-deserved tribute he shares when describing the selfless, loving dad we were all blessed with—and loved beyond words.

CHAPTER THREE

Unexpected Relocation

"Before you start to judge me, step into my shoes, walk the life I'm living and if you get as far as I am, just maybe you will see how strong I really am." — Sayingimages.com

"How can people be so heartless, how can people be so cruel, Easy to be hard, Easy to be cold, how can people have no feelings, how can they ignore their friends, Easy to be proud, Easy to say no, and especially people who care about strangers and social injustice, Do you only care about the bleeding crowd?"—Extracted from some of the lyrics of "Easy to Be Hard", in the musical "Hair"

With the look on Eddie's face when he arrives home from work today, my years of experience visually reading his feelings tells me, immediately, that something is wrong. Apparently his, and most of his department's Informational Technology positions, are being outsourced to countries that will provide the same work skills for much lower salaries. Essentially, without warning, he is out of a job. Impulsively, I throw my arms around him and tell him everything will work out, sounding more convincing than I feel. The truth is that while many other families are also in the same situation, affected by the outsourcing, the majority of them have two incomes—while my current medical conditions prohibit that. At the moment, I feel insecure considering this recent unexpected development, especially while paying for our girls' college educations—but at the same time, I want to be supportive and positive for Eddie.

With the I.T. market drying out in our state, showing optimism is getting more and more challenging, however. Even expanding his search to surrounding states yields no positions to apply for within his expertise. After two months of bills piling up, with no meaningful income, we're faced with taking more dramatic steps. Finding and applying for a job listing that fits his qualifications— over a thousand miles away—unfortunately becomes a "no-brainer". Through technical telephone interviews, he is offered the six-month consulting assignment. Though financially relieved, the degree of compromised health currently challenging me is physically overwhelming, especially with the untimely responsibility of having to quickly pack two season's worth of clothing—and prepare to apartment hunt. While I can't afford not to, I question where I will find the strength this abrupt, (but necessary), move will require.

With virtually no choice we head South, passing through many quaint and inviting towns along the way. Doing my best to focus on something other than the regret I feel having had to leave family, friends, the familiar lifestyle I'm accustomed to and practitioners and medical facilities I utilize for overseeing my disconcertingly still unresolved health status, I turn to the beautiful scenery—trying to convince myself that maybe this won't be so bad, after all. Eddie and I discuss how it will be an adventure—one that we're embarking on during an opportune time in our lives. With Stacey married and Storey in college, they are adults themselves—secure living independent of us, (while at the same time knowing we're only a phone call away and/or within a short plane flight if needed). Just as I am buying into my own magical thinking, a huge city with at least four lanes approaching it comes into our view—along with signs that leave no doubt we've reached our destination. I don't know what I was expecting—but certainly NOT this! Rather than the Southern charm I'd always heard about, it seems wherever we stop is reminiscent of the hustle, bustle of New York City. What HAVE we gotten ourselves into—and why is it I'm wishing we were in one of the many lanes exiting this metropolis rather than entering it?

Over a meal at one of the best Italian restaurants I've ever been to in my life, (and I've been to a lot!)—where the waiter suggests we share a softball-sized meatball, (no exaggeration), with our pasta and salad entrées—we strategize. Finding a place to live is the priority, only trumped by checking our travel-weary bodies into a hotel as soon as possible.

Refreshed from a night's sleep that nothing could have interrupted, including noise, bed comfort, etc., we head to a realtor who shows us several locations in the upscale area Eddie's assignment is in. The problem we note right off is that most require a longer--term lease than we're looking for. Frustrated, we eliminate one potentially doable place after another until we're finally able to convince the owner of a gated condo complex to allow us a shorter commitment. Relieved, we sign on the dotted line of a six-month lease. Next, we select enough large furniture rentals, (couch, bed, television, etc.), to get by—and then purchase a new mattress at a chain bedding firm and small necessities from a local wide-variety department store. Eventually entering our hotel room, we're exhausted from a long but fulfilling day. Tomorrow the rental furniture will be delivered, allowing us to move into our own place.

Dropping Eddie off in our shared car, I give him a hug and wish him luck on his first day—while I continue on to the condo where I wait for the rental furniture to arrive. When he comes home, it is to the previously stark unit we rented transformed into a cozy, temporary living space. The smile on his face as he walks in tells me my efforts were appreciated.

Eddie is enjoying his new assignment as well as the co-workers he is interacting with. In addition, we find ourselves taking full advantage of the beautiful, warmer–than–New England climate we are accustomed to at this time of year—allowing us to participate in more outdoor activities, than usual, at the end of his work day. The restaurants are amazing and from the looks of the scale, I'm probably frequenting them far more than I should!

To prevent the isolating feeling an unfamiliar place such as this could encourage during the daytime, while he is at work I pursue activities at the local church we attend—as well as community art exhibits, plays, tours, etc. Within weeks I've also made many new friends and, immersed in such pleasurable distractions, before I have time to think about it his assignment is over and we are back home—where he is fortunate to be recruited for a local I.T. consulting position. Life is good!

As if a warning not to become complacent prematurely, I rhetorically ask myself who overheard that positive thought—and found it necessary to demonstrate otherwise. Attempting to navigate a large department store, challenged by my blurry vision, I feel like one of Pavlov's mice avoiding roadblocks everywhere I turn as I head for the prescription counter. First, a child unexpectedly darts in front of my shopping cart as her mother quickly yanks her to safety. The fear reflected back at me from the mom's eyes is genuine—as is her disgust in how close I came to hitting her child. Her unspoken message is clear—had she not done that, this seemingly unaware adult, who is stumbling through the store like someone who has just imbibed in a liquid lunch at a local bar, could have injured her unsuspecting toddler. As I attempt to apologize, her stare transforms from understandable concern for her little girl to unmistakable anger directed toward me. Storming away with no acknowledgment of my effort to say "I'm sorry" for something, unlike the scenario she probably projected on the movie screen of her mind—the one that showed a woman who was intentionally careless in avoiding her child—was out of my control. As she does, I'm frustratingly reminded of the misjudgments, in association with disabilities, made by others who have no firsthand exposure to them.

My next "obstacle" is the elderly gentleman using a cane who stops short directly in front of me—with no warning—to ask his wife's opinion of an item. Fortunately, I am able to take the brunt of the awkwardness it results in by tipping into one of the shelves next to me, sparing him while at the same time hurting both my pride and my shoulder. It is with a sigh of relief when I'm finally done checking out and on my way to the car.

As though just what the doctor ordered, my eyes sting with appreciation when I arrive home and open today's mail, touched by words that reflect in-depth understanding only firsthand experience could express. Converting intimate thoughts straight from her heart into written words that she could share by mail— penned on a multi-colored, floral-embossed thinking-of-you card—a recently injured close friend divulges her newfound, (but temporary), reality. Discussing how healthy she was until now, her note reflects the shocking transformation an activity-altering injury, which occurred a week previously, has had on her life. Interpreting what she says, I can almost visualize the stalactites and stalagmites in my brain crystalize into a rationale healthy people employ when dismissing those who are not. Her words, which describe a newfound empathy for what she refers to as a "small fraction" of what my life must be like, indicate that until now she—and many others without physical challenges—couldn't begin to comprehend. Truthfully, they don't have to. As much as we like to think of ourselves as totally loving and compassionate individuals, to a degree we all dismiss or compartmentalize realities we'd rather not face nor allow to clutter our minds. Despite the misfortune of others, our lives should—and do—go on. Often, it is not until, (and if), a similar circumstance hits home that we truly empathize.

In "Invisible Illness and Friends Who Don't Get It: What to Do", by Lisa Copen, she states, "If you live with an invisible illness, you may find the emotions of coping with peoples' doubts about it can be harder to manage than the disease itself. Most of us with chronic illness must eventually accept our condition. In order to live our best life, we need to educate ourselves about the disease and make well- researched decisions about treatment."

Unfortunately, it doesn't end there. Most of us can identify, firsthand, when she continues: "But we have no control over our loved ones when they choose not to accept our illness or sometimes even acknowledge it. Their skepticism can last a lifetime and damage our self-worth and many relationships."

Indisputably, there are patients who can identify firsthand with premature dismissal, unkind remarks, etc., (myself included). I know what it is like to see friends I love—(many of whom I thought of as my most dependable support system)—deny a reality I cannot—and the hurt it resulted in is indelibly imprinted in my heart. The brave front I tried to project the first time I went out socially after discharge from Neuro I.C.U. following my brain bleed, (to be discussed in greater detail later in the book), wasn't brave at all— inside I was scared and insecure, unsure if I was physically strong enough to pull it off—terrified that my shaky, unsteady legs wouldn't hold me and that I'd fall in front of everyone, or worse, that I could have another bleed and be ambulanced back to the stroke center—potentially not as fortunate this time. There are no words to describe how much I needed the hugs I longed for that night—but indifference I didn't understand, (and I still have difficulty comprehending), prevented—at least from some. Suffice it to say I found it unconscionable to have the kind of brain bleed from which many people die, without any concern and/or acknowledgment, from a small but important minority whose blatant lack of compassion shocked me.

Equally awkward for me was pretending to have a good time with people I knew well, as my swallowing was compromised around the lump that formed in my throat the first day I showed up on oxygen and a walker. Ignoring the equipment as though it didn't exist, without as much as an inquiry as to why I needed it or how I was doing, sent a strong message that didn't require words.

I can further identify with the author's sentiments when I am told, in no uncertain, angry words how frustrating it is to the people around me that I never get better. Part of me wants to scream, "Do you think I like it? Can't you see that I am doing my very best to live a full and productive life, balancing health challenges others have found easier to remain bedridden from? But the reality is they cannot. While intellectually they know the meaning of the word "chronic", they are bored with the longevity of this disease. (I don't blame them—so am I!) The unfortunate truth, however, as Lisa Copen points out—(and just the thought of which, in terms of someone I love being effected, makes my eyes fill), is that there is a high probability that at some stage in their lives everyone will experience their own health challenges—(hopefully on a considerably reduced level)—at which point they will have a better understanding of what a chronically ill friend's life is like. My prayer is that everyone reading this book can learn through my words—not by firsthand experience.

What troubles me most, however, is the degree to which skeptical reactions of others influence misdiagnosis. As a result of the severity of their illnesses being unacknowledged and/or misinterpreted repeatedly, does the self-esteem of such patients dip so low that they become emotionally paralyzed—finding it easier to agree—(while disconcertingly aware the dismissive theories presented are incorrect)—rather than challenging their physicians' suppositions? If so, this is a sad commentary contributing to why the statistics for misdiagnosis are higher than they should be—but certainly one that can be addressed through more active listening and recognition of the fact that not only do diseases present atypically in different patients, but there are so many rare ones—far too many for any medical professional to commit all their symptoms to memory.

But, in my opinion, that isn't the most important consideration here. The priority should be realizing something is going on and researching it beyond one's experience background, if necessary. Not every patient in desperate need of treatment, who walks into a physician's exam room, does so with a readily identifiable condition. THAT DOESN'T MEAN IT ISN'T REAL OR THAT INTENSIVE, (possibly even life-saving), TREATMENT ISN'T REQUIRED! Though not responsible for all medical errors that inflate misdiagnoses statistics to the unacceptable levels reported, I'm convinced that until this reality is realized and acted upon more aggressively, they will be higher as a result.

CHAPTER FOUR

The Best of the Best—Or Is It?

"You may be the only person left who believes in you, but it's enough. It takes only one star to pierce the universe of darkness.

Never give up." —Richelle E. Goodrich, "Smile Anyway"

Like a pillow unintentionally ripped open during a stress-releasing pillow fight at a slightly insecure teeny-bopper's first sleep-over, (and night away from home), which, in my mind is nowhere near as effective as popping bubble wrap—and a lot messier—a blizzard of flakes blankets our world. Unlike the feather storm however, this blizzard is real and, under normal circumstances, no one in their right mind would be out traveling in it—unless, of course, they'd just been offered another patient's cancelled slot at one of the most highly regarded diagnostic medical facilities in the country—one which it seems like I've been waiting forever to get into.

Determined not to miss what we pray will be a life-saving opportunity, the fact that we cannot book a flight at this late notice does not deter us. Eddie didn't hesitate in the least when I called him at work to relate this unexpected, last-minute opportunity. According to his naturally good sense of direction, he assures me that by driving most of the day, with a few hours factored in for sleep, I will be in plenty of time for my 6:30 A.M. appointment. While he closes up shop and leaves work early, I contact hotels near the facility. Because most evaluations are done primarily on a day-patient basis, the institute is situated in an area surrounded by them—in some cases adjoining the enormous medical campus. After a twelve-hour ride that, due to the inclement weather took longer than it should have, we unceremoniously flop onto the invitingly irresistible bed in our hotel room. Unfortunately, Eddie only has the luxury of a few hours of sleep before having to make the long trip back to work.

Dropping me off at the hospital the next morning, our glistening eyes betray the mixed emotions we both share. Spoiled as I've been, a foreign insecurity flows through my veins and envelops my whole being, as we say good-bye at the massive clinic entrance. While in the past his work schedule allowed the flexibility, (except in very few cases), for him to accompany me on these critical diagnostic searches, with I.T. assignments now in such competition it is getting more and more difficult. Further, having exhausted all of his vacation days primarily on previous nationwide medical excursions, unfortunately they are no longer an option.

A hug that seems just a little tighter—and lasts a little longer—is tell-tale evidence of how hard this estimated five-day separation will be for both of us. Yet, the reality of having so much riding on a diagnostic consult at one of few facilities I know of that is so respected for their success in identifying and appropriately treating what were initially labeled "mystery illnesses" at previous hospitals, helps put things in perspective for us. Just knowing this consult could have a positive—even potentially life-saving outcome—makes it worth it to both of us.

Despite this shared optimism I will myself to focus on, it is with much trepidation that I enter the overwhelmingly huge facility— my long list of pre-scheduled appointments with physicians in multiple specialties I have yet to meet—(but with whom I've already established an emotional trust, just by being here), in hand. Saying a silent prayer that this is the right decision, I reference the first doctor's name and suite number from the top of my list and attempt to navigate my way to the appointment.

While I will be the first to admit I'm both directionally and technologically challenged, I never quite realized to what extent until now. I have no clue where to begin, which set of elevators to take, (as not everyone stops on all floors), nor what wing I'm supposed to be in. Fortunately, momentary signs of panic, (including wet palms and a dry mouth), ease up with the discovery that there are multiple information booths strategically located throughout the sprawling, high-ceilinged main floor. The absence of others standing in lines in front of the stations, however, serves as a demeaning indication that not every patient is equally sense-of-direction challenged—not to mention fighting the urge to lose their breakfasts at the realization that, at the moment, I appear to be the only one. How am I EVER going to get through this week, I ask myself, expecting no answer—and, not to be disappointed, getting none.

Despite the reassuring advice dispensed by the attendant at the booth "crutch" I depend on—that I will make my appointment on time—I'm doubtful and insecure once I'm on my own. Looking around the massively-impressive lobby, I'm overwhelmed. The blurriness that compromises my vision renders the signs difficult to read, especially in conjunction with vertigo damage that challenges my balance by tipping me to the right. Eventually, with an audible sigh of relief only I can hear, I locate the office of the first specialist I'm scheduled to see at the end of a long, sparsely-decorated, but tastefully modern-designed corridor.

Sitting in the filled-to-capacity waiting room, my eyes self-consciously dance from cluster to cluster of people. Though uncomfortably conspicuous, I can't stop. You know that feeling when you find yourself intrigued to the point of almost involuntarily staring—but quickly looking away to avert the attention of your subject should he glance in your direction—almost a guilt response? Awkwardly, my curiosity trumps guilt as my eyes continue to dart back and forth throughout the waiting room. As they do it occurs to me, through this admittedly envy-producing visual, that everyone else is accompanied by someone—in some cases, several people. Before I have time to lament on how much easier this week would be if only Eddie could be here, my name is called—and my whirlwind week begins.

Following a woman dressed in cheerful, bright-pink-colored scrubs, whose kind face is overtaken by a flushed, sheepish look as she apologizes profusely for mispronouncing my last name, I'm led to a small exam room where she verifies my current medications and records my vitals. She then explains that my initial visit is with Dr. Bevins, an internist whom I'm told will oversee my care during the entire evaluation, regardless of how many other specialists are consulted. Based on the results of various interviews, scans, blood work, and other medical procedures, he will determine any additional tests that should be considered and/or doctors I might benefit from seeing, scheduling them accordingly.

If it were my choice, considering the presenting symptoms, I would have opted for a rheumatologist as the coordinating physician—but it is not. "So, suck it up and be grateful that there was an opening for you at such a prestigious and reputable medical facility", I silently admonish myself. Besides,

I haven't even met this internal medicine specialist—shouldn't I at least give him the benefit of the doubt?

My thoughts are abruptly interrupted by a knock on the exam room door, followed by the entrance of a white-coat-clad man with distinguished professional attire peeking through from underneath— whom I correctly assume is Dr. Bevins. Immediately put at ease with his warm demeanor and welcoming smile, he further ensures my comfort by initiating an ice-breaking conversation referencing my long trip to the facility—not to mention the blizzard that accompanied us. After sufficient time for introductory pleasantries is expended—and with the lack of hesitation of someone experienced in doing this many times before—he smoothly transitions from small talk to a serious discussion regarding why I am here.

Methodically, he notates every one of the more than twenty symptoms I describe, occasionally asking for more specific clarification. By devoting considerable time to the history taking portion of our visit, he offers me the opportunity to give uninterrupted detail to what I'm experiencing. Impressed with his listening skills, which he demonstrates by accurately summarizing what I reported when I'm done, I'm also appreciative that at no time does he make me feel rushed, which is a refreshing contrast to a few physicians I've seen in the past—especially one who, watching the clock on his desk with eyes darting back and forth, tennis-match-like, distracted my concentration as he monitored the length of our visit. Refreshingly, Doctor Bevins is just the opposite. By not even accepting calls from other physicians, he makes me feel like a priority during this reserved time slot—and I must admit, it feels good.

During the physical exam, which is much more thorough than most, he discusses the statistical chances of my leaving with a diagnosis. Am I really that naïve? It never even occurred to me that I could leave this renowned medical center without an answer! Yet, disconcertingly, according to him a significant number of patients evaluated do—no closer to diagnosis than when their marathon medical week began. The desperation only a scared, life- threatened, untreated patient can appreciate wants to pretend this isn't true—but knows, firsthand, (as the annoying lump in her throat even further corroborates), that he is right. Once again, I'm forced to face reality: medicine is NOT an exact science. Frustrating as it is to hear, I respect physicians with the integrity to admit they don't know what is wrong as opposed to some who insist their diagnoses are beyond question, despite indications otherwise. Based on my own personal experience, as well as that of several other patients described later in this book, I'm convinced such close- minded thinking is inarguably responsible for at least some percentage of the excessively high misdiagnoses statistics.

While Dr. Bevins continues, imparting the potential for leaving without a diagnosis—which I was unprepared to hear—age-inappropriate little girl magical thinking, that I will leave the hospital "all better", is replaced by a more adult, realistic scenario— resulting in a quick but sincere silent prayer, that I'm not in the undiagnosed bracket discharged without an answer.

Continuing, Dr. Bevins describes the next group—those that are not definitively diagnosed, but for whom there are symptomatic treatments that considerably improve quality of life, as the search for an answer progresses. Though more appealing than the first category, I'm selfish—that's not enough for me! I want to leave here with a name and description for whatever has made my life hell over the past few decades—and I want to share that information with a few friends, relatives, physicians and acquaintances who contributed to it by not believing me. Most importantly, I want to save my life, which I have no doubt is currently in jeopardy—being consumed by an internal, raging monster that has yet to be identified by me and/or the medical community.

As the optimistic remainder of patients who leave diagnosed is described, Dr. Bevins adds a few more specialists to my list, the size of which already competes with that of a greedy little child's requests to Santa Claus—only I'm not a child, and the consequences of my wishes remaining unfulfilled are far more devastating—much as children may disagree.

Agenda in hand, my hour-long appointment with Dr. Bevins concludes and I leave encouraged that, despite leveling with me about not everyone evaluated here leaving with a diagnosis, (which I respect him for doing), he has a plan in mind—and feels confident as to what additional physicians I need to consult. Reassured by his compassionate and, from what I can tell, encouragingly optimistic attitude, any former hesitation having an internist in charge of my case is gone.

What a difference three floors and a long hallway to an adjacent wing can make! Unlike Dr. Bevins, the eye specialist, Dr. Grayson, doesn't have a warm, fuzzy bone in her entire body. Entering the room, she makes absolutely no eye contact as she reaches for my records on a nearby table. (To be honest, if I were a guy, she wouldn't know as she never looks at me!) Immediately uncomfortable with the dismissiveness this cold, impersonal physician demonstrates as she asserts that according to my chart my vision is fine, I feel my face flush heatedly with anger. Frantically retrieving words from the personal thesaurus in my mind, I grasp for any persuasive enough to convey the distorted and impossible-to-label-normal vision I've struggled to see through since the "bubble incident"—yet, I fall short. Nothing I say impresses her concern. Approaching me to conduct an exam, it is the first time in the fifteen minutes I've been here that we make eye contact—but my gut tells me this is nothing but a superficial formality. Her dismissive attitude is unmistakable. At the conclusion of the least comprehensive eye exam I ever recall having, she summarizes our session by reiterating that my eyes—the ones whose distortedly blurry vision struggle to discern the large EXIT sign above the door—are perfectly fine, all the while charting—and never once looking at me again prior to leaving the room.

Though momentarily stunned, I ask myself why, as brain cells that store negative memories—(the ones we all have, whether we choose to admit it or not—and would prefer were erased)—kick in. Unable to escape the involuntarily resurrected reminder that this isn't the first situation in which I've encountered such undeserved dismissal of real physical symptoms, in the privacy of my thoughts I ask myself how many other "Eileens" there are in this world. As though answering my own question, it occurs to me that if the personal accounts other patients have shared with me are any indication, there is no doubt why misdiagnosis statistics are so unacceptably high.

Frustratingly, there is nothing I can do, at least at the moment, to address the unprofessional way in which I was just treated. Emotionally drained, I decide to take advantage of the twenty-minute break before my blood work appointment. Sitting in a coffee shop I'm a little overwhelmed reviewing the remaining schedule for today and the rest of the week. There are sleep studies, nerve-conduction tests, various scans, chest x-rays and a myriad of other tests. Like a college student cramming a full semester into a one month, accelerated Summer session—in order to earn their degree in an ambitiously condensed period of time—my schedule leaves little opportunity for much else, including bathroom breaks—speaking of which, I spill the remaining half a cup of coffee down the drain as I rush off to find a ladies' room.

Whomever designed this complex didn't have a clue as far as what it is like to navigate with disabilities. While I give them credit for the wide-open spaces enabling ease of movement for wheelchairs, walkers, crutches, etc., the massive campus with appointments scheduled at opposite ends—allowing so little time to get from one doctor's office to another—is a disabled person's nightmare!

Eventually arriving at the blood lab, (two information desks later), I'm sweaty and out of breath—but, amazingly, on time. Immediately apparent from the crowd of bored and/or apprehensive faces in the waiting room, rushing was unnecessary. Taking a seat, I hear several easy-to-pronounce last names called, one-by-one. As a phlebotomist comes out stammering over the next name on her pile of charts, I know it is a good sign. Standing up, I ask if she is looking for me. Appreciatively, she thanks me for "rescuing" her from trying to pronounce it and takes me into a room where she draws more tubes of blood than I've ever had taken. While she does, I silently pray that at least one will elicit a diagnosis.

Exhausted, physically and emotionally from a long and draining day consisting of additional forms to complete and appointments to fulfill, I head toward my hotel room which, though adjoining the hospital one must traverse through a confusing maze of mall-like stores before reaching it. Too tired to even consider eating in one of the many restaurants I pass along the way, I grab a sub from one of the fast food stands and take it back to my room.

Once there, I barely have the energy to sit up and eat, instead slouching through half of the sandwich while leaving the rest for another day. Much more enticed by the steaming hot bathtub water that beckons my muscles, I submerge appreciatively into relaxation and pain relief beyond description. While the aching in my legs succumbs to the therapeutic heat hugging them, I reflect on the events of the day. Excepting the eye specialist appointment, today was indicative of a promising start. Having pre-reviewed my schedule for the rest of the week, I'm most interested in tomorrow's rheumatology consult. Convinced I'm experiencing a form of vasculitis, my hope is that they can confirm if it is—and, more importantly, treat it effectively.

Suddenly startled when the alarm goes off at the ungodly hour of five A.M., I'm momentarily disoriented. In my sleepy stupor, I lie in bed confused by the darkness—wishfully hoping against hope that it's really Eddie's alarm, summoning him for work. Reaching over to nudge him to stop the incessantly squawking, purposely louder-by-the-second, obnoxious—(but effective)—clock, reality awakens me completely when my hand is met by an icy cold sheet on the empty side of the bed. Disconcertingly, he's not here—and the alarm is for me.

Oh, no, I've been to the information booths so often the attendants are beginning to recognize me! Embarrassingly, they inquire as to whether I found specific physicians' offices I'd asked directions to yesterday—but today is another day, with lots of new locations to explore—(and information kiosks I haven't exhausted yet)—so here goes!

Coming as no surprise that the sleep lab is far from the other offices, given it is most conducive to sleep if located in a remote, quiet area, I'm relieved to find it so quickly—actually impressing myself by arriving a few minutes early. As the technician scrapes my scalp to apply electrodes, I'm concerned when he explains I have only forty-five minutes to sleep. Considering I've just awakened and don't feel in the least bit tired, how accurate and diagnostic will this test be if I can't magically make the sandman reappear? As suspected, he doesn't and the technician is unable to trace sleep patterns, as hoped.

Disappointed with what I'm convinced was a predictably wasted test, (wouldn't it have made sense to instruct the patient not to sleep a certain number of hours prior, or to schedule it much later in the day?), I leave with some of the glue residue still in my hair, despite the tech's best efforts to remove it. Wearing a dark shirt, I'm self-conscious of what looks like copious dandruff, as the dry flakes coat it like snow falling during a February blizzard. Any embarrassment quickly dissipates as the irony of my concern is trumped by a strong dose of reality: here I am having my brain scrutinized for abnormalities and I'm worried about looking as though I have dandruff! On the other hand, some distraction at this point might be healthy, considering it could be overwhelming to focus exclusively on the potential negative findings from an intensive evaluation such as the one I'm undergoing.

Sitting in the rheumatologist's office at my next appointment, I find him welcomingly pleasant and unmistakably thorough. What concerns me is his inability to connect the symptoms I describe with a specific diagnosis. My doubts regarding his experience with the condition I present are confirmed when he admits, with humble honesty, that what I am relating is far beyond his expertise— initiating a call to the department head for a consult. (Dripping with respect for this physician who demonstrated more concern about securing an accurate diagnosis for his patient, than assigning one himself—that he wasn't certain of—I await the arrival of the doctor he went to summon.)

The soft-spoken, immediately-likable rheumatologist he introduces me to is considerably older and unmistakably more experienced, judging by the content of detailed questions he adds to those I'd been asked previously. Based on my responses, he concludes that the symptoms appear more neurological than rheumatological. Frustrated, I leave feeling like a football passed from one doctor to another, only unlike each team longing to get their hands on it, I don't get the impression that any specialty wants to take responsibility for my case. Just yesterday I was evaluated by neurology—who told me I needed to be seen by rheumatology! In fact, they were the ones to add rheumatology to my list of appointments, when unable to explain my symptoms. Understandably discouraged, a sinking feeling manifests in the pit of my stomach with the realization of what I accurately predict I will hear at tomorrow's "wrap-up" visit with Dr. Bevins—no diagnosis found.

Sitting alone in my hotel room, tired and missing Eddie, it depresses me to think this long, arduous and expensive trip was for nothing. More importantly, I am no better off—physically—than the day I arrived. As a tear escapes and rains down my cheek, I dismally contemplate my future, (or lack thereof), if some doctor doesn't figure this out soon.

As expected, Dr. Bevins has no explanation for me, other than that I fall into the category of patients who leaves this facility undiagnosed. Delivering this message with compassion, he leaves the door open for further follow-up should additional symptoms develop. As we shake hands, I know in my heart I would never feel confident returning if this week of extensive testing couldn't elucidate a diagnosis—(not to mention to have been subjected to one specialist who refused to acknowledge my symptoms existed!). Fortunately, that did NOT reflect the attitudes of the others I was sent to. There is a HUGE difference between not knowing what a patient has—(and being humble enough to admit that)—and not believing there is something really going on because you, personally, can't readily diagnose it. The eye "specialist" I saw has much to learn from her far more professional peers!

Praying to God to guide me regarding what to do next, I buckle my seatbelt and the cab driver starts the meter, heading for the airport.

CHAPTER FIVE

There's an Answer Out There Somewhere—and I'm Not About to Stop Searching Until I Find It!

"The most common way women give up their power is by thinking they don't have any." —Alice Walker

Frustrated with my lack of diagnostic success, particularly neurological, out of desperation I resort to my own research—discovering the name of one of the most well-credentialed and impressive neurologists in the country. Immediately calling the contact number provided, in the hope that she is more experienced with the type of symptoms with which I'm presenting—than those I've consulted previously—I listen impatiently to the entire menu as instructed, before selecting a prompt because "their choices have recently been updated". (Haven't they all?) Unarguably skeptical that almost every specialist I see managed to change their system at the same time, (with recordings practically identical to the one I am now hearing), before I have further opportunity to stew over what I consider an unnecessary delay, I'm directed to punch in number three to be connected to a receptionist in charge of making appointments.

When scheduling my first consultation, I'm informed that the neurologist only sees patients who have been evaluated by her assistants, (not physicians), prior to the specialist's appointment—a protocol she adheres to for all subsequent visits, as well. I suppose that dependency, in itself, should raise a red flag—but I'm desperate enough to overlook a policy I might ordinarily question if it means seeing a physician with experience impressive enough to possibly solve these inexplicable neurological events. With that in mind, I make my first appointment(s).

Optimistic and relieved that the long-awaited day is finally here, neither the far-too-early-to-be-awake time we need to be at the train station, nor the doctor-is-running-behind explanation discourages me. Truthfully, the anticipation of finally getting some answers and more importantly, effective treatment, exhilarates me and makes the time pass quickly. Before I know it, a staff member leads us to an exam room where she proceeds to take my vitals.

Just as she releases the pressure of the tightly pumped up blood pressure cuff, one of the assistants we were told to expect to see prior to the specialist appears—a warm smile defining her face as she pleasantly introduces herself.

Conducting a typical medical history inquiry, my responses are detailed and accurate. I describe where and how I hurt, when the symptoms started, what brings them on and a myriad of other specifics. Comparable to a job interview, I am cognizant of how much every answer counts. The difference is that far more is at stake than a position—we're talking about a life and what I say matters—"big time"!

Objectively able to look past her pleasant personality, I'm unimpressed with her medical "expertise" as she tells me, during a neurological exam, that her findings are "normal", in this decidedly NOT normal body! However, instead of letting my discouragement with her lack of diagnostic abilities get to me, I silently reassure myself that when the specialist I came to see evaluates me, she will uncover far more than her superficial findings and inaccurate assessment, not to mention dismissive summarization. Swallowing hard, it takes every ounce of determination to respect and listen to my logical brain cells as they kick in, challenging the illogical ones that tempt me to impulsively tell her how wrong she is. Miraculously succeeding, as she exits the room to summon the physician we came to see, the one we never met but somehow already have so much faith in, I silently pray our confidence in this new doctor doesn't prove unfounded.

Before entering the exam room, we can't help but overhear the very inappropriate and unprofessional way in which the staff member—whose voice we, by now, recognize—loudly converses outside the door, within our earshot, (and undoubtedly that of others'), conveying personal patient information. Detailing familiar symptoms, it doesn't take a rocket scientist to realize the patient she is describing is ME! Dismissively, she predispositions the neurologist by telling her I look fine and that my neurological exam was completely normal, causing Eddie to roll his eyes in knowing disgust, hearing the grossly unimpressed evaluation he has heard far-too-many times. While it takes every ounce of restraint to activate hidden determination I didn't even know lived within me, to ignore the anger that inflames my body with the heat of a severe sunburn, I resist the temptation to walk out—hailing the first cab back to the train station. My skin prickling with discouragement from head-to-toe, my rational side kicks in, reminding me that I owe it to myself and my family to give her the benefit of the doubt, (I think!).

Entering the exam room, the physician introduces herself and proceeds to regurgitate the same unimpressive summarization we are now hearing for the third time; once during the assistant's exam, next within earshot of a discussion outside my door and now the exact words of someone else spurting out of the mouth of another. Unable to explain why I am experiencing such "events", as she also labels them, she decides that the best way to capture one is to admit me, once again, to the hospital for four days of consecutive video EEG monitoring—this time at her facility. While still cognizant of the bad taste the last tethered admission test left in my mouth, on the other hand we're encouraged that she is willing to investigate my symptoms further. Somewhat surprised, but in no way disappointed, a bed is available within a week for EEG testing at the hospital where my specialist has practicing privileges. Optimistically, packed bag in hand we board the train headed to the distant institution where, finally, we hope to get some answers and, more importantly, resolution to these scary, inexplicable symptoms.

To ear-piercing screeches rendering the conductor's voice non-discernable, thanks to an inferior public-address system, passengers are otherwise distracted as he attempts to announce various station stops. Some sleep contentedly, mouths wide open as they drool onto their freshly-pressed work attire, too deeply anesthetized by the sandman to feel embarrassed. Observing them, I'm reminded of the innocence of childhood—a time in life when people are much more real and less inclined to care what others think. Certainly, if someone took a picture of most of these sleeping adult passengers and showed it to them when they awoke, they would be mortified—but just for this limited period of time, that is not their concern—and there is something comforting about that.

Other passengers chatter incessantly. Some discuss social activities, while many strategize about work assignments. The majority are using some type of electronic device, playing games they have considerately silenced so as not to interrupt others.

Despite all the chaos that fills the narrow cavity of the train car, engulfing commuters with stimuli from every direction, I'm too absorbed in today's up-and-coming admission to be completely distracted. Before long, we are at our destination, a fact I'm aware of not from the incomprehensible announcement the conductor makes, but from the large identifying sign above the station.

The efficiently run admission process evidences how often their well-trained staff has registered new patients. Within an hour of arrival, I'm in my private room, (which is mandatory for EEG's at this particular facility), and being interviewed by a nurse. (What medicines do you take? Do you have any allergies? Have you had any surgeries? etc.). As I complete my responses to the same questions I've been asked repeatedly over the past month, usually by various staff members at the same office, I'm told the repetition is due to the fact that their peers used a different screen when they recorded the identical answers.

All too soon, the time I've been dreading arrives. Eddie needs to leave in order to catch the train for his long ride home. After all, if we have any hope in keeping up with my astronomical medical expenses and associated out-of-state travel costs, someone has to work! Much like with the last admission, despite knowing I'll see him in less than a week, glassy, begging–to-spill pools of moisture reflecting at him as we say good-bye are physical giveaways of how much I'll miss him—body language that no matter how brave a front I attempt to demonstrate fails to conceal feelings involuntarily resurrected from deep inside, housed in a place I mistakenly thought only I could access.

Before I can further lament his leaving, I'm distracted

by an EEG technician who enters, explaining he is going to glue multiple leads to my scalp so that colored monitoring wires can be attached. (Silently—but not naïve enough to mean it seriously—I entertain the thought that I've had this done so often I could probably put them on myself.) Though the glue has a potent chemical odor that unpleasantly takes up residence in my nostrils, and the process is time-consuming, as with previous EEG's nothing is painful. Approximately forty-five minutes later, my wired headdress is complete and a gauze sleeve is wrapped over it to prevent the wires from disconnecting when I sleep.

Like a prisoner in solitary confinement, I am only allowed—except for bathroom breaks when the wires are disconnected from a main wall outlet (which I am immeasurably grateful for)—to move within the parameters of how far they reach, which is about two feet beyond the sides and foot of my bed. Trust me, these four days can't pass quickly enough for me!

While in the middle of attempting to consume a typical hospital-style dinner, (do they all have stock in lime gelatin?), my physician and another one of her many assistants walk into the room, providing me with a socially acceptable excuse to place the insulated cover back on my uneaten meal, never to be taken off by these hands again.

Following some small talk about whether I find my temporary home away from home accommodations comfortable, my doctor introduces me to the newest staff member accompanying her and then informs me that she, like the physician in charge of my previous hospital EEG admission, is planning to wean my seizure medications for the duration of my stay—in the hope of triggering an event that can be witnessed and recorded. Within the short time it takes for this recommended protocol to traverse from her mouth to my ears, icy chills of fear pulsate through my veins, initiated by recollection of the visual deterioration this discontinued medication resulted in previously. Unable to hold back, I nervously share my concerns regarding what happened when this was last done— which she is sensitive to. The difference this time, according to her, is that I will not be subjected to the extreme deprivation that was employed previously. The decrease in medication will be gradual—the goal not being complete exclusion but just enough to encourage seizure activity, which sounds safer and more reasonable to me. With the assurance that should I report any visual changes the original dose of medications will immediately be resumed, she then writes out the drug adjustments she discussed with me, hands them to the nurse and leaves the room with her assistant closely behind.

Absorbing myself in one of the crossword puzzles I judiciously packed in preparation for what I knew from experience would be a long and boring stay, the time passes quickly and before I realize it bedtime is here. Exhausted from our two A.M. wake-up time to catch the train, the sandman owns me at the moment—but not for long. Groggy but aware enough to check my watch, it is just after midnight when I awaken from hustling and bustling noises in the corridor. An alarm sounds as staff members run into the room next door. Someone is crying. In an apologetic voice, between sobs, a woman keeps saying, "I'm sorry". My guess, from what I overhear, is that she soiled herself during a seizure that set off her room alarm and initiated immediate staff response.

Much as I would like to say it is unintentional, the human side of me knows otherwise as I eavesdrop intently to the compassionate way the multiple responders reassure her. Demonstrating more kindness and understanding than if both emotions were on steroids, it is immediately apparent that this isn't the first time the experienced staff encountered a comparable situation. With ears that have no business listening, I'm in awe as I hear them transform the focus of an understandably embarrassing event into something positive.

Pointing out as they get her cleaned up that what just happened is a good thing—because they were able to capture a seizure and, as a result, now know the specific type she is having and how to treat them, they end on an even more encouraging note, enthusiastically giving her the news that since they have all the information they need, she will be discharged tomorrow.

Lying in bed trying to get back to sleep is an effort in futility. I'm too wound up. Instead, I put on my light and take out a crossword puzzle. Fortunately, I brought several because if tonight is any indication of what to expect during the rest of my stay, I'm going to need them!

Within a half hour, my head begins to ache and my limbs involuntarily jerk—forcefully enough to hurt. Additionally, there is a gurgle-like fluid sensation emanating from my throat that I not only feel, but hear. As they manifest, I vaguely recognize them as symptoms I've had in the past—but so long ago, prior to starting seizure medications that lessened their frequency and intensity so dramatically, I'd almost forgotten how severe they used to be—until now. On the rare occasions that I don't remember to take the drugs, the slightest symptom intensification acts as a reminder of their return—allowing me to discourage them with appropriate medications long before they reach the uncomfortable stage they are at tonight.

Though previously they didn't scare me, after the incident I inadvertently, (though, as it continued, somewhat purposely), just "witnessed" with my ears, I'm emotionally paralyzed from fear that the same thing could happen to me. Despite the goal of admission being to capture a seizure, now knowing what can occur during one has chilled my feet to ice. Before I can put my "worry brain cells" through further stress activation, the sandman overpowers them, magically shutting my eyes as I drift back, appreciating that the remainder of the night is uneventful. During morning rounds, my physician reports that some abnormal brain waves registered on my EEG recordings, ones that she can't explain but find intriguingly questionable. Assuring me that they will probably materialize into an identifiable diagnostic answer before I'm discharged, she exits my room.

Listening to the woman in the room next to me elatedly converse with the nurse, I can hardly believe she is the same person I overheard last night. Excitedly preparing for discharge, one would never know she experienced a serious seizure just hours earlier. Instead, she very coherently discusses the medication changes her doctor ordered and a few minutes later a wheelchair is rolled into her room by a staff member who escorts her down to her car, where her husband is waiting.

My mind swimming with confusion, I don't know whether to be envious or relieved. Envious because she knows exactly what she has and can leave after a one-night stay, or relieved because I didn't experience a scary seizure like the one I heard far more of than my ears deserved to be privy to.

The next few days remain consistent with yesterday. My limbs jerk forcefully, the headaches continue, and, in addition, with the decreased seizure medications I've begun to drool—profusely. Yet, despite waking up multiple times a night from a drenched face uncomfortably sticking to a soaked pillowcase—in conjunction with the other symptoms—no measurable seizures are captured. Because of the unlikelihood that they will be if they haven't been by now, I'm discharged four days after I was admitted.

Though one of my sons-in-law offered to accompany me from the hospital to the train station, (a kind thought volunteered due to an assignment nearby), I see no reason to imposition him when I am perfectly capable of getting there myself. After all, it isn't as if I had surgery. Confident in my decision, I hail one of several cabs strategically located in front of the hospital's semi-circle-shaped, covered main entrance. As the driver lifts my suitcase into the trunk, I fasten my seatbelt and, once he is behind the wheel, ask to be driven to the train station.

It takes no more than a minute after he drops me off to realize the mistake I've made in "going it alone". Insurmountable weakness and fatigue I wasn't expecting compel me to desperately search for any available sections of the cold, smooth, marble train station walls to lean against on the way to the platform.

Regretting my too-late-to-take-back decision, I clumsily struggle to the track identified in overhead letters so small they are almost unreadable—the one that corresponds to my destination. As I do strangers approach me, kindly offering to carry my small but difficult-for-me-to-negotiate suitcase. If this isn't evidence to this sometimes too-proud-to-accept-help woman, that I'm not the only one aware I've misjudged how unable I am to pull this off, independently, I don't know what is! One gentleman, with a grandfatherly-like kind, compassionate face responds to my refusal of his offer of assistance by warmly pointing out, "This is what we are here for, to help one another". Curtailing my reflection regarding how true that really is, the train pulls in and to my relief, the closest available seat is just steps away—to which I appreciatively drag my suitcase and ungraciously plop down with an audible sigh—which I am surprisingly not even self-conscious about. The only thought on my mind is that I'm finally on my way home!

Excited as I am to see Eddie at our local train station hours later, where I all-too-willingly relinquish my suitcase, grateful to have him wheel it to the car, my enthusiasm is bittersweet. Yes, I'm discharged and back home—but not with any answers or, more importantly, resolution—and it shows.

Very early the next morning, (3:00 A.M. to be exact), I lie awake in our dark bedroom, unable to sleep from deep, penetrating pain in my head and at the base of my neck. Between the metronome-like ticking of our nearby alarm clock and Eddie's peaceful and rhythmic breathing, for the past several hours I've been the solo audience to a symphony only I hear—one to which my thoughts seem synchronized. Unlike the serenity one would ordinarily associate with such innocuous noises, I'm fearful as I lie here considering every possible scenario that busy daytime distractions thankfully allow me to partially escape—whereas, relatively speaking nighttime quiet refuses to interrupt. Unable to sleep, I snuggle into the protective comfort of the crook of Eddie's warm, outstretched arm where, many unnerving thoughts later, fatigue overcomes worry as I eventually drift off.

What seems like only moments later—and actually is—I awaken to rapid, involuntary rhythmic tapping of one finger against the mattress. Even in my now-conscious state, it is somewhat surreal—like watching a children's toy that has been wound up and has to complete its cycle before stopping. Nothing I do interrupts the continual tapping as I observe this weird phenomenon in sleepy, blurry-eyed disbelief. The unsettling part is unlike the toy that traverses across the floor until it runs out of steam, requiring it to be wound up again in order to move, I did nothing to initiate the tapping—nor can I stop it. Even scarier, it isn't coming from an inanimate object—it's attached to me!

Within seconds, the tapping which awakened not only me—but Eddie as well—ceases as suddenly as it began, with both of us falling back to sleep. Minutes later, the process repeats itself, this time with a different digit affected. Life is frightening and uncertain, while rest is sporadic at best, and so my night, like most others, goes—with several more similar interruptions. Yet, when I describe these episodes to my current neurology group, once again they are downplayed with descriptions like “itty-bitty irregularities here and there”. Excuse me, but I don’t think so! I refuse to accept this explanation—would you?

CHAPTER SIX

I Have a WHAAAT?

"It is during our darkest moments that
we must focus to see the light." —
Aristotle Onassis

Understandably discouraged by the recent diagnostically unrevealing hospitalization, my desperation to be heard—with the degree of seriousness the severity of this condition requires— escalates. Just when I feel I don't know how much more I can tolerate, or where to turn next, a new level of overwhelming pain takes up residence in my body. Hoping against hope that the lease it signed is a short-term one, the fierce headache accompanying It is so all-consuming it comes close to disabling my ability to think. Fortunately, before it does I'm cognizant enough to realize I'm falling. Quickly grabbing the top of my dresser, I catch myself seconds before my knees would have hit the floor.

Sweating profusely, my hands trembling noticeably, I somehow manage to have the presence of mind to call my gastroenterologist, a decision which I have no doubt confuses readers, given my symptoms. Initially, he wondered why as well. Explaining that the severe headache was instigated by straining in the bathroom, I further clarify any confusion by informing him that I've had it ever since—admitting in a scared, shaky voice that I'd also vomited, (gross as it may sound), what looked like a tablespoon of grey pudding. Finally, thinking it important, I share that I took an adult- strength analgesic.

Instead of reassurance, his honest voice-of-experience response worries me more—as if I wasn't concerned enough already! Telling me it is not my G.I. tract that he is concerned about, but my head, I'm instructed with unmistakable conviction—from a voice I've come to trust, (and can't ignore)—to get to the Emergency Department immediately. With that, our conversation ends just as Eddie walks into the house following a round of golf. Talk about good timing!

With the headache not only persisting but slightly increasing in intensity, I quickly update him as we head to the hospital. (Writing this, I can almost picture the crease-lined brows of concerned readers, admonishing me in words I can't hear but know they are thinking, questioning why I didn't just call "911"—I guess I have no good answer other than to say, in retrospect, I realize I should have).

Arriving at the hospital, I detail the incident to the triage nurse. It doesn't take a rocket scientist to realize the severity of my situation, based on how quickly we are taken back to an exam room, (even before these bodies are afforded the opportunity to begin to warm chairs in the waiting area). How often does THAT happen in busy Emergency Departments?

Without delay, a physician's assistant enters the room and questions what occurred as a nurse takes my vitals. Even in my headache-induced, confused state of mind there is no missing how impressed the P.A. is with my symptoms—and not in a good way. His questions are very specific and my responses eye-opening, based on the expressions this terrified patient can't miss staring back at her.

Perhaps the answer that peaks his interest most during the history taking portion of my visit is what I say in answer to his question, “Is this the worst headache you’ve ever had in your life?”, to which I nod my head up and down, (until I realize doing so only magnifies the pain). I now understand where the expression, “I can almost see his wheels turning” came from, based on the look of consternation on his face. Trust me, if brains had wheels, his are spinning out of control!

Ordering a head C.A.T. scan, he returns within minutes after it is administered. With a stricken look on his white-as-a-ghost face, he enters the exam room and shuts the door. “You’re not going to believe this”, he says in a somewhat stuttering voice that indicates he almost doesn’t, himself, “but you have a brain bleed. We’ve already sent for an ambulance to transport you to a hospital where the best neurosurgeon in the state is currently located”.

His words turn my mouth into The Sahara Desert, fear absorbing every droplet of moisture, leaving my tongue like sandpaper. Ambulance? Neurosurgeon? Brain bleed? It’s too much for me to process. Clinging to Eddie’s hand, my dry mouth struggles to coherently enunciate the words, “I’m scared”, to which he responds, “I’m scared, too”. He really doesn’t have to tell me; fear that registers in eyes I’ve known and read for more than four decades says it all.

Before I have time to absorb the unexpected and shocking news I was given only minutes ago, two paramedics enter the exam room with a stretcher. While strapping me on it they query as to whether I get sick on rides, warning me that this is going to be “the ride of my life”. (Hmm, literally?) Somewhat intimidated by that possibility, this non-ride-lover admits to it—immediately after which I’m given anti-nausea medication.

Listening to the ambulance attendants warn Eddie not to try to keep up with them, as he heads to the hospital, causes the gravity of my situation to manifest within me in an even scarier way than it had before. Too much is happening too soon for this to be anything but extremely serious—and the hand I need to hold most isn't available at the moment—instead, in another vehicle, preparing to steer itself to the hospital—with the driver as terrified as I am. Trembling uncontrollably as I stare up at the rapidly moving hospital ceiling, (more accurately, the rapidly moving "me")—being transported to the ambulance, I'm not sure if I'm more afraid of the known or the unknown. Not certain of what to do, I turn to the most reliable source I know of to get through challenging situations—prayer.

As I'm wheeled by the nurse's station, I can hear the staff buzzing about the patient with the brain bleed, selfishly wishing it were not me they were talking about. Apparently one nurse recognizes me, blurting out, "Oh my God, I didn't realize it was YOU!". In my confused state of mind, even though I must know her, the face matching those words is unfamiliar to me. Before I have a chance to give it any more thought, I'm loaded into the ambulance and we are on our way.

As EKG leads are attached and blood pressures are taken, I try to distract myself from the seriousness of the situation. In doing so, I notice the ambulance has a musty odor to it, much less sterile smelling than I would have expected—and that the quarters are so confined the attendants can barely move within them.

Try as I might, distraction attempts prove ineffective when the paramedics radio the hospital every few minutes with the update "still alert and oriented". What does that mean, I worry silently, as I struggle to swallow what now seems like a ping pong ball sized lump in my throat.? Do they anticipate that I'm going to lose consciousness or, at the least, become unable to respond coherently to their questions? Despite my current challenging medical state, the efforts they are making to ascertain that I remain awake and aware are impossible to miss, including being queried repeatedly as to my name and whether I know where I am.

Before my preoccupation with what is going on inside the ambulance can continue further, I'm amazed to learn that we've reached the hospital. If I had any doubts, they dissipate immediately when the doors to the ambulance fly open and I'm given a stretcher ride that doesn't miss a bump. Surprisingly, during my about-to-become-nauseated transport to the Emergency Department, I'm actually cognizant enough to realize the impressive way the paramedics shout out important medical data (acquired during the ambulance ride), to the staff. It is delivered quickly and efficiently within a few minutes, after which their critical job is done and they head out.

Understandably, Eddie has not arrived yet, obediently and wisely heeding the warning not to try to keep up with the ambulance. By the time he does walk in, I'm hooked up to more monitors than I care to count. Additionally, I'm given several basic exercises to test my current thinking, including what is the president's name, do I know what day it is, where I am, etc.

Various scans and tests are ordered, including an arteriogram, in which a camera-loaded catheter is threaded up to the brain, allowing an interventional neuro-radiologist to determine if there is an operable cause—like an aneurysm—for the brain bleed. In my case, there is not.

Grateful not to require neuro-surgery, my condition remains critical, given the bleed is in my brain. I'm admitted to the Neuro Intensive Care Unit for one-on-one monitoring. My vitals are closely watched, as is the size of the bleed—the hope being that it stops on its own.

In a way, the entire experience is surreal. So much has occurred in a few short hours. Suddenly I'm sitting in an exam room desperately holding the hand of the love of my life, while looking at a face that appears to have aged thirty years from the stress of today's news. Lines of fear crease his unusually pale forehead, while his eyes jump from monitor to monitor, much like a tennis ball during a match—only Eddie's look is not that of an interested and excited spectator—but rather of frightened and unmistakable disbelief.

Attentively clinging to every word he utters, Eddie reminds me of how strong I am and how much I've fought already, encouraging me with reassurance that I will get through this, too. If only his words matched his body language, but they don't. Nothing in his demeanor convinces me that he believes any part of his well-intentioned, wishful thinking inspiration—nor do I.

After several days in Neuro I.C.U. we're relieved to learn my condition improved enough to graduate to the step-down unit, where I remain for further monitoring before being discharged.

Sitting in the exam room of my neurologist, whom I've returned to for the first time since the brain bleed, I'm a little put off when one of her assistants congratulates me for finally presenting with something "clinically measurable—neurologically". Continuing, with something I interpret between a smirk and a smile, accompanied by a voice that indicates little concern, she remarks that I've now "earned my badge". As she does, I can hardly believe what I am hearing. To me, this is NOT a joke. I must admit that a few choice words for her, some of which I wouldn't find appropriate to print, consume my thoughts at the moment. How DARE she minimize the "bubble incident" which occurred over a decade ago, by labeling the brain bleed as my first measurable neurological incident? More importantly, how could the neurologist she works with not give more credence to that previous event that changed my life, irreversibly? Further, what compassionate and professional specialist would congratulate a patient who'd just had a brain bleed by saying she'd "earned her badge"? NOT acceptable!

Understandably, my confidence in this particular assistant, who exhibits more dismissiveness than the severity of my symptoms justify, continues to dissipate. Further, it frustrates both of us to learn that when providing an update to the neurologist, (keeping in mind I am not allowed to report my symptoms firsthand), she neglects to mention an important finding discovered while on a three-week heart monitor. We, and my cardiologist, think it is significant that every time I documented a neurological event it was preceded by an irregular heartbeat. Convinced this omission was too meaningful to ignore, Eddie looks intently at the neurologist and asks why that is happening. Her initial response is to circumvent the question with a silent, darting and surprised look in the direction of the assistant, who blushes with embarrassment as she utters an awkward, "Oops!" (Excuse me, but I've just had a brain bleed and reported what could amount to a significant clue as to why, one she neglected to share, and all she can say is "Oops!" I think not!)

Sitting on the hard, inflexible metal chair, I uncontrollably see the in silence, processing what just took place. To verbalize what I'm thinking at the moment would get me thrown out of the practice, which, given the way I've been dismissed might not be the worst thing to happen, but where would I go?

By reputation, this physician is one of the best. Can I afford to lose her, even though part of me wants to scream, "No wonder medical mistakes continue. If only you took the time to see your patients with unresolved medical issues, especially complicated ones, EXCLUSIVELY, rather than relying on the observations, assumptions and opinions of less experienced, (though inarguably trained) professionals, maybe there would be less "Oops" and earlier and more accurate diagnoses".

Due to her inability to diagnose me to date, my next visit with the neurologist results in what Dr. Edward Rosenbaum reveals in his book, "A Taste of My Own Medicine", a technique medical students are sometimes taught to employ when they can't come up with a definitive answer—think psychological. To my silent annoyance, because I know what I'm dealing with is physical, (but can't yet prove it), she tells me she is scheduling psychological testing. Unfortunately, to object would mean losing her as a neurologist and I'm confident that my life depends on having one.

Due to a rare cancellation, there is an opening today for the three-hour test, allowing us to avoid another long train trip out-of-state. Asking if I mind my husband being present during the interview process, I immediately agree to and welcome his presence. When the psychologist and the student she is training begin by asking whether he has noticed a change in my personality lately, I find myself wondering who is being interviewed—him or me. His answer is automatic and unhesitating—that I am the same person I always was. They then ask if he observes any up and down mood swings, which he does not. Following a few inaner questions, he is sent to the waiting area while the mentoring psychologist exits the room, leaving me to complete the evaluation with the student.

Beginning with configurations of blocks, we move on to replicating pictures I am shown in advance—which are then removed, repeating a series of numbers, identifying common items, etc. On several occasions, I find her soft mumbling difficult to understand, having to ask her to repeat herself, (which is later negatively documented in her report). How subjective does it get? Do you mean to tell me the patient is at fault when the interviewer speaks too quietly or incomprehensibly to be understood? Think again! This is how misdiagnosis occurs.

The verbal portion of the test reminds me of being back in school, taking an exam I'd prepared well for—only this time there was no studying involved. During the puzzle segment, I wish there had been, though I doubt it would have helped. My ability to see relationships between some of the more challenging ones is virtually non-existent.

Before I have time to lament my potentially undiscovered learning disability, (and/or residual stroke damage), the test concludes and the mentoring specialist returns to join us. As I'm bending over the desk to sign a release of medical records form, the psychologist asks me how long I have been married, to which I respond, "thirty-nine years". Appalled and in shocked disbelief by her lack of professionalism, my ears can barely process what they hear next, as she whispers to the student, "She's not wearing a wedding ring". Intrigued by the importance she places on this observation, given not all married couples have rings, I look up just as she is pointing to her ring finger, silently mouthing to her student, who didn't hear her, "No ring". (Excuse me, but isn't this the same person who notated that I didn't hear HER during my exam?) Stunned silent, while understandably annoyed, I stubbornly decide there is no way I intend to pull my necklace, from which my engagement and wedding rings dangle, out of my shirt, (where it had slipped inside). Had they done their homework, they would know that fingers can swell from Behcet's Disease, but that's not the issue. The unprofessionalism and judgmental attitudes displayed by those in a field respected for its objectivity is inexcusable! To surreptitiously signal and whisper to an associate, in the presence of a patient, tells me more than I care to know about this "specialist" and leaves me wondering if the wrong person underwent psychological evaluation. In addition to never being able to recommend her, I highly question the competence of a physician who could. More importantly, once again it is situations like this that encourage misdiagnosis statistics to escalate.

Stammering uncomfortably at my next visit, as she reads my psychological test results, the neurologist tells me she knew they would be normal and they are. Looking more fidgety by the minute, she goes on to say, (or cover up for the unnecessary exam she demanded I take), that she was just trying to establish a baseline when ordering it. Yeah, right! She was looking for a quick explanation for a diagnosis which, to date, eludes her. Rather than take responsibility for not knowing what was causing the symptoms, (which is very understandable—certainly doctors aren't expected to recognize every rare disease that exists!), the onus was initially on the patient to prove the situation was physical. In order to do so, I was required to undergo hours of multiple tests, irrespective of how difficult this was to do while so very ill. The questions that come to mind are what recourse do patients have in situations such as this—and when will rare diseases be considered and explored in far more depth before resorting to psychological assumptions? It is as difficult for patients in this frustrating, undiagnosed position, (even more so, because they are the ones challenged by daily untreated symptoms), as it is for doctors who can't label their illnesses. However, failing to aggressively pursue, to the fullest extent, the possibilities of PHYSICAL diseases responsible for these "mystery Illnesses" only assures further misdiagnosis.

Disgust and fear riddle our conversation on the train ride home. There is no doubt in either of our minds that I am so ill I can barely function attempting to live through every challenging day, yet once again, I've just dismissively been told I have "little bits of irregularities here and there". Like a closet stuffed so tightly with clothes that one has to literally pry each hanger out when selecting an outfit, my mind can't fit another adjective to describe my condition other than those I've already shared with the medical community.

Months later—but physically just as sick—we again embark on a train during the wee hours of the morning, headed for a follow-up office visit with my neurologist. Even the long eight-hour commute doesn't discourage us—if anything, we're looking forward to this particular appointment more than usual, knowing the entire visit will be exclusively with the physician rather than primarily with one of her assistants, all of whom she relies on far too much, in mine and Eddie's opinions. From what I understand, there is a conference out of state that all assistants will be attending and therefore won't be available for office responsibilities today.

Optimistic as I am when we arrive, disconcertingly less than two minutes into the visit I am forced to blink my eyes, repeatedly, trying to discreetly hide the tears begging to break out of their anatomical jail—threatening to spill uncontrollably, exposing my no-longer-possible-to-hide private feelings to the world—or at least to the doctor I'm too proud to share them with. The unexpected sting of an emotional slap in the face causes me to reel, inwardly, from the uncompassionate words I never would have predicted I'd hear. Though not physical, the pain—on a totally different level -is just as real.

In spellbound disbelief, we listen as the physician describes in a voice dripping with annoyance—only matched by the irritated look and body language she displays—how frustrating a patient I am to doctors. (Hmm, let's think about this. Do car mechanics lash out angrily at customers who bring in automobiles with problems that aren't easy to diagnose and fix? How about plumbers who, after multiple attempts, can't stop a leak? In my opinion, if they do, they're in the wrong profession!)

Continuing on, the doctor informs me of the exact number of patients in her practice, disgustedly pointing out that of them all I am the one to walk in with the most concerns. In an attempt to respond, I utter one syllable before she immediately interrupts me, sarcastically demanding that I only report a single symptom. Noting what must be a very bewildered look reflecting back at her, she says, “You can’t do that, can you?”, with a knowing, uncompassionate smirk enveloping her countenance. When she again insists that she will only listen to one symptom, I have a real dilemma. Do I tell her that my G.I. specialist, who contacted her on my behalf, believes, (as do I), that I am having abdominal seizures which require aggressive treatment or do I ask her if the nocturnal urinary incontinence I experienced since I last saw her could be DUE to a seizure? Opting for the possibility of some relief from the doubling over abdominal events, I describe the episodic ascending waves of stomach pain that occur repeatedly throughout the day and night—while intentionally omitting, as per her request, (demand), a serious symptom I have no doubt she should know about.

Questioning me further as to what my G.I. specialist thinks is going on, which is confusing to me as I know they consulted by phone, (but later learn was a rushed conversation indicative of little concern), I share that he believes the vagus nerve is involved. Throwing her arms up in the air, she dismissively responds that the vagus nerve is related to almost everything.

Sitting back further in my chair, which, unlike those in her other exam rooms which are made of uncomfortable, ungiving metal, I can feel my back create its own impression into the soft, supple cushion—much like a young child preserves a handprint his parents will covet, forever, in Plaster of Paris. The difference is that I don’t want to save the memory of this or previous visits to this office any longer—nor do I plan to continue making such “memories”.

As though I needed any further convincing, (which, at this point, I certainly do not!), the neurologist tells me, with the most uncompassionate delivery possible, that the seizures I’m experiencing multiple times a night, arousing both of us, "aren't going to kill you". Ending with a sarcastic and dismissive, "Do you get the point?", as a matter-of-fact I do, (my mind answers with words he can't hear)—only not the one YOU are trying to make!

In her well thought out article, "9 Signs You Should Fire Your Doctor", by Angela Haupt, senior editor of Health at U.S. News, she lists the following reasons:

1) You don't mesh.
2) Your physician doesn't respect your time.
3) Your physician keeps you in the dark.
4) The physician doesn't listen.
5) The office staff is unprofessional.
6) You don't feel comfortable with him, or wonder about his competence.
7) He doesn't coordinate with other doctors.
8) He is unreachable.
9) He is rude or condescending.

In my current relationship with this particular physician, numbers 1), 4), 5) and 9) stand out unmistakably bolder than the others. 1) Clearly, our interaction is challenged. I feel limited and/or absent one-on-one time is dedicated to her patients; instead, leaving that to other less experienced staff members whose interpretations are sometimes respected, unquestioningly, by the doctor—to the point that mistakes are not always recognized. 4) My physician demonstrated her lack of listening skills on more than one occasion, but never as blatantly as when she arrogantly, in-my-face demanded that I report only one of several symptoms I'd traveled hours to discuss with her. Should it really be the patient's responsibility, medically untrained as she may be, to determine the most critical symptom to report? I think not! 5) In my decades of pursuing diagnoses, having seen over one

hundred physicians prior to finally being diagnosed with Behcet's Disease, a segment of this latest neurologist's office staff demonstrated the most unprofessionalism I've ever encountered. Whispering in a patient's presence, in order to transmit a misjudgment on their part—to another staff member—exhibits immaturity inappropriate for employment in a medical facility. They should be ashamed of themselves!
9) Rude and/or condescending treatment is unacceptable on EVERY level. No more than a patient should be disrespectful to her physicians, neither should her doctors be to her. Mutual consideration, in my opinion, is one of the most effective foundations for good doctor/patient relationships. With the majority of physicians encouraging such teamwork, there is no reason for patients to subject themselves to those who do not.

As difficult as being assertive enough to make this decision was, I have a far bigger dilemma—where do I go from here? One physical challenge after another serves as an unsettling reminder that I can't do this on my own. Waking up to my left hand flip flopping rapidly, alternating as it slaps the bed from palm to the back of my hand, further corroborates that reality. Ironically though, as I watch the involuntary movement so nonchalantly, I momentarily question if my unconcerned reaction is normal. Wouldn't someone else be scared if it were happening to them? From my perspective, the frequency of these episodes, occurring daily—for years—cause me to be somewhat immune to them. I suppose if I allow myself to focus on the possible frightening ramifications they might represent in the future, it can get overwhelming. Instead, I welcome the denial that kicks in to protect me from doing so. Yet, my denial must be incomplete, given the questions that silently materialize in my mind—deep, but unfortunately not deep enough to ignore. Much as I'm almost afraid to pursue answers to them, the logical cells in my brain remind me I must. Healthy bodies don't wake up nightly from episodic, rhythmic tapping. What other words can I possibly use to convince my doctors of this? More importantly, how do I stop this unwanted energy emanating from inside me, manifesting itself in so many scary and undesirable ways? This can't go on—or can it? And, if it does, will I?

CHAPTER SEVEN

A Scary Incident—Questionably Diagnosed Depending on Which Consulting Physician is Asked

"The Best Way to Predict Your Future is to Create It."

—Abraham Lincoln

Sitting in a local diner shining with fifties-like chrome, our reflections ricocheting back at us from fingerprint-free mirrored walls, one almost expects waitresses to take orders on roller skates. If my long-term memory is accurate, (and to-date, I believe it is), the only thing compromising the authenticity of what I believe is modeled after the interior of metal trailer-like diners I recall visiting as a child, (now modernized on the exteriors while maintaining the memorable indoor charm), is the nonexistent juke boxes—with numerous songs listed on pages made of stiff aluminum that one "read" by turning a control dial on the top. Teens fortunate enough to have the required coins to play their favorites often selected the same song—over and over again—much to many diners bored distress. As my mind reminisces back to the bobby socks, saddle shoes and poodle skirt days my older cousins introduced me to, I'm grateful places that resurrect those warm family memories still exist, which is probably responsible for why I suggest this nostalgic location so often.

Today is no exception. Seated next to, and across from, three friends I frequently meet for coffee—in a soft, comfortable, vinyl cushioned booth—we joke that we are here so often, in the same seats we automatically gravitate to, that the establishment should reserve them for us—with our names engraved on brass plates. But this morning, which seems quite normal except for the headache I woke with and can't seem to shake, is about to prove to be no joke.

In the middle of a funny story I'm telling relating a silly dream I had last night, my thought process is suddenly interrupted in an unnerving way—with the realization that the friend sitting directly across from me starts to disappear from my vision, progressing from blurry to all grayed out, to nowhere in sight! Why is it that I feel she hasn't gone anywhere—and if anyone is exiting this planet to some unknown place, it's me—not her? Confirming my supposition, I hear her laugh at the story I continue to tell—challenged thinking aside. Relief flows through my veins, relaxing me like a pre-surgical sedative, at the reassuring discovery that she is gradually re- appearing within my vision.

Considering I'm seated on the inside of a well-padded booth surrounded by friends, I feel a sense of security—enough to elect not to mention the incident, which none of them are aware of yet. Before leaving an hour later I nonchalantly mention to one friend, out of necessity, (because we had made plans to walk immediately after breakfast), that I decided to postpone our well-intentioned exercise until another day. Big mistake! She missed her calling—she should have been a detective. Knowing me so well, she is immediately suspicious—aware I wouldn't renege without a good reason. As the incessant "grilling" continues, I relent, explaining that though I'm fine now, I'd just experienced a scary episode about an hour ago—which surprises her because she was completely oblivious of the event.

Offering me a ride home I decline, given I'm only a few minutes away and feel confident driving. Suspecting to some extent it's false bravado, (a truth I silently admit only to myself), my suspicions are corroborated by the sense of relief I'm overcome with when within sight of my soft, supple, over-stuffed recliner. Though inanimate, the somehow knowing empty cushions entice me with a silent, irresistible invitation to mold my tired, overwhelmed body into its conveniently available soft leather hug—an offer I can't, (nor want!), to refuse. When what seems like every muscle I own relaxes as it defines its impression into a semi-permanent memory— like a child enveloped on all sides by a bean bag chair, it's a "no brainer" that this is where I intend to spend the rest of the day. Comforted by an embrace I long for but my working husband won't be home to provide for several hours, I effectively and artificially create a temporary one myself, wrapped within the welcoming confines of suppleness my currently present dream chair affords. As I do, I reflect on how fortunate I am that the frightening, all-too-familiar brainstem stroke symptoms this incident resurrected, disappeared.

My relief is short-lived, however, when my friend returns a few hours later to see how I'm doing—and so do my symptoms. Once again, I elect not to share my fears, though during her entire visit I'm ever conscious of the E.R.-worthy intensity of my current escalated condition, which remains frightening and undeniable to me. Besides an atypical tingling of my lips, there is an unmistakable pulling sensation in the corner of my eye. The minute she leaves, I rush to the bathroom mirror. The subtle but disturbing revelation that reflects back transforms me physically, resulting in clammy hands and a throat as dry as a desert. Sometimes a little knowledge is a scary thing—and I'm terrified. Much as I try to pretend this isn't happening, my contorted, slightly askew lips are unconvincing. In addition, there is a significant drooping of my left eye—one that doesn't take a neurologist to recognize. Coupled with the visual anomalies I experienced just hours earlier, I have no doubt I'm exhibiting stroke symptoms.

In a perfect world, I'd go right to the hospital and request evaluation for a possible stroke. However, through firsthand experience I learned that symptoms like these can—and often do—resolve on their own, leaving the patient feeling like a fool when they arrive at a medical facility trying to describe, in detail, symptoms that are no longer present.

At the same time, too scared to attempt to handle this on my own, I take the safer route and contact my physician's office. Since she isn't in today, I schedule an appointment with one of her colleagues who, fortunately, has an opening. With a degree of common sense controlling my actions, even under these very challenging circumstances, I know enough from the return and increase in symptoms not to get behind the wheel of the car. Consequently, the sound of his key clicking our door from its locked position to unlocked is music to my ears as Eddie enters our condo. By coincidence, and much to my relief, he is home early for his pre- scheduled, annual physical at the same practice.

Arriving at the office, we are each called into our respective doctors' exam rooms. Because I referred to visual problems when I made the appointment, part of my work-up includes reading an eye chart, which appears far more distorted than usual.

Just as her assistant completes recording my vitals the physician enters the room. Taking one look at me, she immediately comments on my askew smile. As frightened as I am during this time when I suspect I'm having a stroke, (and with good reason!), the disconcertingly pathetic thing is I'm also overwhelmingly relieved— relieved that someone beside myself, a respected practitioner in the medical field, is aware of it, too. What a disappointing but understandable commentary this thinking demonstrates, regarding how important such affirmation is—even at a challenging time like this—especially to a patient prematurely dismissed with legitimate and serious physical symptoms in the past. For the first time, the "Do no harm" instruction crystalizes my thoughts in a way it never did before.

During her evaluation, my physician notes that my tongue deviates to the left when I'm asked to stick it out. Of further concern from her perspective, my heartrate is twice as fast as normal, (which comes as no surprise to me—I'm scared beyond words!). Corroborating what I knew when I called, (but prayed was unfounded), I'm having stroke symptoms—right before our very eyes!

In the kindest, most compassionate way possible, even though I sense she isn't as relaxed about my condition as she does her best to portray, she explains what I have no doubt is inevitable—so sure that I packed a bag before leaving home: I need to go to the hospital, immediately—by ambulance.

Despite the fact that I knew it was coming, I'm not prepared, (evidenced by eyes that fill almost—but not quite—to the point of spilling). Unsuccessfully trying to conceal my embarrassment, my quivering voice is an obnoxious give-away, the pitch being several octaves higher than normal when I inquire as to whether I can have Eddie drive me, instead of going by ambulance.

Sensitive to my understandable request, but at the same time determined to convince me otherwise, she persuades me with a firsthand, personal story in which a spouse in a similar situation— though medically trained—decided to drive, when devastatingly, the results were fatal on the way to the hospital. Hearing that, it is suddenly a "no brainer"—I would never want something like that on Eddie's conscience. Without hesitation, I agree to go by ambulance.

As she starts oxygen flowing throughout my body, I ask for my husband, whose physical is interrupted so he can be with me. With barely enough time to hug him and say "I love you", the ambulance attendants arrive and I am whisked out of the exam room.

It is with considerable trepidation that I leave the office of specialists I trust impeccably, to be transferred to the care of hospital physicians I've never met. The last thing I say while being wheeled out is, "I'll be back"—all the while trying to ignore that nagging fear materializing into a question that eats away at me from deep down, at that very personal level of thoughts one is almost afraid to share, (even with herself),—will I be?

Once in the ambulance, it amazes me to observe how much is accomplished before we even leave for the hospital. My vitals are checked and re-checked, an I.V is inserted, nasal oxygen tubes replace the mask provided in the physician's office—and we are off.

Though I request a major stroke center, I'm told it is too far away and that, by law, I have to go to a closer hospital first, with the understanding that transfer to a stroke facility, once evaluated, is an option. Consequently, I'm transported to a less-distant hospital.

Upon arrival, the ambulance staff, (whom I thought was nothing less than incredibly impressive), speak with voices of experience and urgency as they provide a specific and accurate history, in as few words as necessary to convey all pertinent information—while running alongside of the gurney to the curtained E.R. bay pre-reserved for me, as they do. Anything they don't volunteer is quickly answered in response to the hospitalist's questions. After transferring me from the gurney to a much more comfortable hospital bed, they wish me good luck and are on their way.

The nurse assigned to me is so kind and compassionate that I'm not even impatient or frustrated when she asks me the exact same questions I just answered all morning. Do both sides of your body feel the same? Any numbness? Double vision? Headache? Tingling?

My response to her question regarding how long I've had symptoms elicits a reaction that makes me uncomfortable—and a little scared. Learning I've had them for eight hours, it is impossible to miss her unmistakable wincing, as her lips curl and her eyes squint. In a caring voice, she asks why I didn't come in sooner—to which I'm not quite sure how to reply. Deciding to go with the most honest answer, (which, given the severity of my symptoms, sounds dumb even as the words slide off my tongue and into the receptive ears of the by-now understandably curious nurse), I explain, "I wanted to be sure my symptoms would be considered clinically significant before coming in"—my skeptical voice betraying me as a patient whose authenticity has been challenged in the past.

"Are you kidding me?", the silent voice that makes all of us second guess our actions, asks. As a patient, I shouldn't even know the phrase, "clinically significant", much less have to be concerned about it—but I do, and I am. Not unlike other rare or "mystery disease" patients, I, too, have been sent home from one facility after the next because the symptoms I reported were not readily identifiable in terms of a specific, (and more commonly seen), disease. As my hesitancy to report stroke symptoms as early as I should indicate, I will do anything to avoid the demeaning stings from these emotional slaps in the face that still resurrect in memory banks I wish I could erase. At the same time, it is a wake-up call to me that by doing so, I could be risking my life—the irony of which is that, to–date, I've expended so much energy just to save it! My nurse's empathy upon learning the catch 22 I've been in is undisguisable.

Noting the same askew features my doctor documented, she pages neurology. After less than the extended wait I'm accustomed to at hospitals dealing with emergency and unpredictable situations, a neurology resident examines me and recommends admission on a stroke watch.

My mistake, (which I'll detail later), is to request transfer to a stroke center for observation. Complying, I'm transported by ambulance to the closest one. Feeling every bump along the route that is currently under repair, the EMT apologizes profusely as we near the stroke center—while I think to myself I can only hope these are the only "bumps" I'll encounter along MY road.

Arriving, I'm immediately unimpressed by the demeaning way in which the big, burly triage nurse treats the unmistakably dedicated EMT. As he shoots a glance in my direction, reporting the askew smile, she asks impatiently and with undisguisable attitude, "Was it visualized?", to which he responds that in addition to myself, (which elicited a skeptical, unconvinced look from her), my physician observed it. It is not until she learns that a doctor saw it that it is documented in my chart.

As the patient, I feel insignificant when it comes to the lack of credibility I'm given in regard to recognizing and reporting this symptom. Fortunately, my personal physicians witnessed and documented it while still present, (before subsiding about eight hours later). But what if they hadn't? Even at that, I feel dismissed—particularly when a doctor enters the exam room, listens to my chest and, after remarking that my heartbeat is very rapid and irregular, minimizes it with the explanation, "probably just anxiety due to having come from a hospital where you were told you were having a stroke". Really? Let's back up a moment. I have a history of stroke. Doesn't it make more sense to err on the side of caution—rather than dismissiveness?

With a nonchalant attitude, I suspect he would never accept from a physician evaluating someone in his own family presenting with the same symptoms, I'm told that I probably had a seizure, (which leave not only myself, but the seizure doctors I contact subsequent to the incident, doubtful), and sends me home with the computer-generated protocol distributed to all seizure patients upon discharge. One of the warnings it includes is not to drive until receiving clearance from my personal neurologist. Given it is the weekend, I will follow the instruction by contacting him on Monday. Though I regret this is the case, I'm discharged from the E.R. feeling no more physically secure than when I arrived.

On the ride home, I'm weak and dizzy—but unconcerned, attributing it to the fact that I wasn't allowed to eat for the past 18 hours—nor was I given anything before leaving. Curiously, even after I resume regular meals once home, it is disconcerting to note I'm still lightheaded and woozy—an anomaly that continues the entire weekend, as does the headache.

With my vertigo intensifying every time I roll over in bed, awakening me from nausea, I'm convinced my body is telling me— in its own language, but one we both understand—that this isn't over yet. As if to confirm my silent—but none-the-less very genuine concern—every blood pressure I take, in compliance with hospital physician's orders, is almost double the low numbers I typically register.

Rule follower that I am, I call the neurologist's first thing Monday morning. Understandably, he is seeing his scheduled patients and not currently available. Leaving a message asking him to call me, the receptionist assures me I will hear from him by noon. When I haven't by late afternoon, I call back explaining I'm looking for clearance to drive. This time she promises I'll hear from him by the end of the day—yet, once again, no call.

With the hands of my clock navigating 24 hours since my finger's first attempt at reaching him by punching in his office number, I wake up on Tuesday morning in that semi-out-of-it state we can all relate to—you know the one that vaguely, somewhere way back in your not-fully-awake mind reminds you that there is something you have to do—but you aren't coherent enough to figure out what. Trying to ignore in-overdrive brain cells as they scramble to solve this nagging urge to remember what it is I'm supposed to do, (as if they weren't scrambled enough by now!), I roll over, wrapping the warm, cozy blanket around me, cocoon-style.

Falling back to sleep, a few minutes after nine I awaken from one of those annoying, computer-generated credit card company calls—the ones that tell you your credit is fine but they just want to know if you want a lower interest rate. Guessing my brain cells must have kicked in during my sleep, I ditch the unwanted electronic sleep-interrupter and remember to call the neurologist's office again. When I do, I explain to the receptionist that I have several physicians' appointments and really need to determine if I have to cancel them or if I have clearance from the doctor to drive. Like before, I request a call from him.

Much later that day, I answer the phone to undisguised irritation in my neurologist's voice, accompanied by a loud sigh preceding his question regarding why I feel unable to drive.

Explaining I was told not to at the hospital, and that the written hand-out I left with instructs me to get his clearance prior to doing so, he becomes condescending, listing the only reasons it is considered medically dangerous to drive—which are few—none, according to him, applying to me. Confused when he mentions seizures among the symptoms that would be prohibitive, I advise him that I was told in the E.R. that I'd had one, which is why I was contacting him. My confidence in his competency quickly dissipates with his, "No one told me about it!"—especially since the nurse advised me my record was faxed to him before I was discharged. But even giving him the benefit of the doubt, if it wasn't, why didn't he request it before contacting me?

In a voice dripping with sarcasm and disagreement, he asks what they based my diagnosis on. Describing my recent symptoms, he concludes that I don't need him—I need a stroke specialist— actually the same stroke specialist who saw me at the hospital and insisted that I see an epilepsy doctor because he was sure it was a seizure and not a stroke! Before ending the conversation in which he tells me there is no reason I shouldn't drive, he also offers to admit me for EEG testing to see if they can capture one of these "events". That, in itself, makes me feel insecure getting behind the wheel of a car. First, he is adamant they are not seizures—and in the next breath he recommends admission to try to capture one!

While "Here we go again—been there done that", clogs my brain with enough too-compelling-to-shake, annoying memories that compromise my thinking, the physical anomalies concern me most—scaring me into pursuing every avenue necessary to resolve them, including multiple opinions. Besides, there is something to be said for being evaluated by a new set of eyes—(I think!).

Taking advantage of the temporary isolation and absence of conversation as Eddie golfs with my brother and sister-in-law the next day, my conflicting, incessant thoughts are all that compete for my attention. As deep reflection surfaces, so do unspoken fears—ones that, though I can prevent from verbalizing, my mind refuses to allow me not to entertain. It is the "what ifs" that frighten me most. What if I awaken paralyzed? What if I become completely dependent and unable to care for myself? What if I suddenly lose my sight? Disconcertingly, a combination of strokes and seizures can cause all of the above.

Fortunately, my rational thinking kicks in and overpowers the negativity, reminding me that no one can predict the future—and that diseases are not necessarily forbearers of serious consequences. After all, perfectly healthy individuals can walk outside and get hit by a car. With restored resolution, I refuse to expend limited energy that could better be used toward fighting this illness than unproductively worrying about the "what ifs"—(until next time!).

Inarguably still insecure and feeling desperate, it is with unshared mixed feelings that I wait on the line while the doctor transfers me to his receptionist to schedule admission for video monitoring, (which will be read by a different specialist).

Politely and apologetically, the voice on the other end—that of the receptionist—explains that the average wait for the few coveted private rooms where monitoring is done is about two months. While scheduling me for the first available opening, she simultaneously lists amenities, including: pristine new rooms with private baths, (which, keep in mind, has shower facilities one can't use while attached to electrodes, regardless of how many days, or weeks, that may be), pull—out couches for overnight family guests, cable T.V. and I'm not sure what else because as she is about to describe the next "perk", she excitedly interrupts herself. Apparently as we speak, a patient calls on another line to cancel, opening up a spot for me only a month away. That works! Immediately reserving the slot before it is assigned to another patient, she tells me she will be in touch before my admission date—advising me to keep an eye out for the information package she is mailing today. With that, our phone conversation concludes.

True to her word, two days later I receive a large package from the hospital. Not only does it include questions I have answered in the past—but several others. Additionally, enclosed is a picture of an inviting, nicely-decorated room—more like one in a hotel than in a hospital—but with the unexpected difference clearly to my advantage, I'm not about to complain!

Filing the envelope away with the intent of refreshing my memory by re-reading its contents again just prior to my scheduled admission date, I absentmindedly forget about it—until a phone call from their office two weeks later, that is. Recognizing the by-now familiar voice of the polite receptionist, she informs me that it is hospital policy to require a psychological evaluation prior to admitting any patient for seizure studies—and, because of that, they'd taken the liberty to schedule mine for the next week.

Though somewhat taken aback to learn of this never-before-mentioned "policy", resulting in a scheduled appointment in which I had no input as far as date, time and/or consent, I can't help but question why neuro-psychological evaluations are protocol PRIOR to EEG monitoring—at least at this institution. At what point does the patient no longer have to PROVE that they are not the cause of their health challenges—but are seriously ill—before more clinical studies are administered? Unfortunately, until the medical profession, as a whole, (rather than the best physicians who already are), is open-minded enough to consider first that maybe THEY missed something clinical—like a rare disease or atypical presentation—misdiagnosis will continue.

Frustrated beyond words, I can almost visualize annoying and incessant splashing as the phrase "Here we go again", swims far-too-familiarly through my head. Taken by surprise, without any time to give thought to this appointment that has involuntarily been scheduled for me, I feel at a disadvantage regarding what to do. At the same time, I can't afford to ruffle feathers and possibly risk being dropped by my neurologist, with no other plan in mind, because I refuse the appointment. Consequently, with considerable unrevealed reluctance, I agree to the time slot.

Some people are really good on-the-spot thinkers, a skill I envy. I'm more the type who, in some instances needs time to assess a situation before making a decision—(which I could've used in this case), rather than agreeing to an appointment that raised a lot of personal red flags. Despite the fact that it may be protocol for the hospital, the more I think about it, the less confident I feel in a neurology practice that looks for psychological causes before investigating clinical. Uncomfortable with a sequence of events that makes no sense to me, I decide to discuss these doubts with my PCP at next week's appointment.

Meanwhile, my negative health changes scare me more than I even dare admit to myself—but can't escape worrying about in the wee, quiet hours of the night, when Eddie's voice is silenced by well-deserved sleep. Unfortunately, even the ticking of the alarm clock—the only noise I hear—is ineffective in distracting me from my inescapable reality. At the same time, the uninterrupted quiet provides a perfect opportunity for some of my best strategizing.

With the video monitoring admission heavy on my mind, objectively I can't help but recognize the value in proceeding with it, especially given my latest episode. What I do have reservations about is the preliminary process involved at the facility where it is currently scheduled. Coincidentally, this hesitation results in a positive effect in that it exercises my brain to the point that it prevents me from sleeping until I come up with a more logical approach to procuring an EEG.

Deciding to go online the next morning, intent on researching other institutions that conduct the same brainwave monitoring, possibly without the same preliminary requirement that I've already tested normal for, I now have a plan—one that allows me the peace of mind to drift off to sleep, no longer negatively preoccupied by feeling I have no input regarding medical decisions associated with my health.

CHAPTER EIGHT

I Can Do Better—And So Can They!

"When one door is closed, don't you know that many more are open." —Bob Marley

Driven by desperation to find a neurologist with the competency and perseverance to recognize and effectively treat what occurred in my brain, seemingly overnight—to disrupt my life so dramatically—I once again spend hours online researching medical facilities and physicians specializing in seizure and stroke diagnoses. By the time my internist's appointment arrives the following week I'm well-prepared, armed with contact information associated with the specialist whose credentials impressed me most. Convinced he is the one I want to see, and with my physician's blessing, I schedule an appointment with the new epilepsy doctor—while cancelling all those previously set up with the original group. Meanwhile, unable to control the worsening vertigo, I'm embarrassed—especially in stores—when I continue to awkwardly and involuntarily fall into strangers, leaving not only myself but the person I tripped into speechlessly surprised—and not in a good way! The longer it persists, the more apparent the importance of this first visit with my new neurologist becomes.

Just like it would be my natural inclination to step out of the path of a drunken person swaying from side to side, I can't help but notice the wide berth the nervous general public continues to provide me. Parents with firm, protective grips on their children's' shoulders intentionally steer them away from me—and understandably so. While I'm mortified by the stumbling and embarrassing lack of balance, at the same time I'm terrified considering every medical explanation I can think of that could be responsible for it.

Fortunately, the day I've been counting the minutes to finally arrive, does. Yet, despite the pleasant young neurologist who greets me and my husband at my first appointment, memories I wish I didn't have—of negative past encounters involving specialists in his field—lead to trepidation, causing butterflies to flutter silently in my stomach, eliciting nervousness that my questionably-convincing smile hopefully shelters from the others. Willing my thoughts to concentrate on thinking positively, I reflect on how it is almost impossible not to feel confident in this state-of-the-art facility. Regardless, like a mom-to-be who feels life for the very first time, and wonders if that is what it really is, I feel the incessant sensation of rippling deep in my abdomen—and question what that sign represents. The difference is that as an expectant mother, I was excited with anticipation when it first occurred, while at the moment I feel too insecure to say the same.

Honestly conveying my frustration with the neurological care received to date, I continue by sharing that if I'm not more successful with his group, my intent—much as I don't want to give up on traditional medicine—is to try alternative approaches. While in my heart of hearts there is no doubt I require regular neurological monitoring and appropriate intervention, CONSISTENT WITH THE DEGREE AND GRAVITY

OF MY CONDITION, I'm not getting it. At the same time, I have no intention of continuing to be dismissed, demeaned, unsuccessfully pacified and/or ignored by neurologists unfamiliar with the unusual presentation of symptoms in my particular case—while unwilling or too busy to research them further. I conclude my part of the discussion by describing the physician whose voice, dripping with irritation, (that her rushed body language confirmed), asked me if I realized how many thousands of patients she had in her practice—and what a frustration I am to doctors because I have so many symptoms affecting my entire body.

The new specialist's raised eyebrows and open-mouthed gape upon hearing this reveal a silently conveyed, but impossible-to-miss, honest reaction. Truthfully, I interpret his less-than-impressed body language as a positive sign. Not only does he hear me, but he is taking what I say seriously. With impressive patience considering my long and complicated medical history, he displays no evidence of rushing me. Actually, sitting behind the closed door of his exam room, there are no interruptions; no knocking, cellphone usage, nor other indications that this time was reserved for anyone else but me. During this vulnerable neurological stage, words can't express the comfort his attentiveness provides, nor the confidence he exudes and transfers to us when he details the specific areas of my brain that have been affected—and, more importantly, the testing he plans to initiate to further elucidate the degree of damage. The treatment options he is considering will be based on the outcome of the scans.

Though I'm not sure why, given nothing he tells us is corroborated by any test results at this point, I'm suddenly overcome by a neurological medical "calm"—one I don't remember experiencing before. He is inarguably the first specialist I've consulted in his field to evoke the same sense of confidence and competence this doctor so humbly does. At the same time, I'm grounded enough to be realistic. What I'm facing is scary—and the conditions he is considering, (which I have no doubt, in addition to those I speculate as possibilities, include potential diagnoses I'm not medically knowledgeable enough to think of)—even more so. However, his demonstrated familiarity with the areas of my brain that are affected and his trust-inducing nature put me at ease as he describes, without hesitancy, the specific scans I need and his willingness to order them.

My silent reflections in deep one-on-one conversation with my mind, regarding this new physician's competency, need to be placed on a temporary hold—rather than distractedly competing as he further educates us through use of a chart that provides a more intensive visual understanding by diagramming the specific nerves involved in the symptoms I report, (in some cases indicating those his office exam corroborated damage to). Immediately skeptical when he tells us I need an MRI/MRA scan of the brain, I can't help but recall the unrevealing ones in the past and share my concerns. My doubts are unfounded after he explains it will be ordered on a newer and higher strength magnetic machine than any I've used in the past. Apparently, this one has the capability of visualizing the brainstem far more precisely. Because machines of this power are more limited than those of lower strength, he gives me the option to travel long-distance for scanning on one of those he is familiar with in his area or to check with various facilities near me to locate a hospital that has one on their premises and schedule it there. Assured it won't affect the outcome, for the sake of convenience I opt for the local choice.

I swear I can literally feel the blood rush warmth to my face with probable premature optimism that this stronger scan, on a machine I didn't know existed, will further elucidate what is going on—and, more importantly, influence treatment in a positive way that improves my quality of life.

So far, I've been unsuccessful in clinically proving the degree of life-changing effects I've experienced since seeing those bubbles more than two decades ago. But no one knows their body better than the person encapsulated within it. Regardless of scans that—to date—don't corroborate what I report, I live, firsthand, in a physically distorted world I do my best to navigate, (because the alternatives are worse!). Repeating the same words I've silently pleaded for years, I pray that this latest scan will be the one that is informative enough to allow doctors to solve my medical mystery— while at the same time the reality that I may have been born too soon for current medical technology interrupts my positive thoughts. Willing my brain not to even entertain that disconcerting possibility I'm afraid to admit even to myself, I utilize my energy focusing on what I've been asked to do next.

Besides the scan, and of no surprise to me, the neurologist wants an in-patient EEG video monitoring study conducted. Unlike at the office in my state that takes the liberty of scheduling psychological evaluations for all patients having EEG's, (without their upfront knowledge), the protocol at this hospital is to order their sleep studies strictly to identify physiological causes—which seems like a far more logical approach to us. The one month wait for the admission I schedule before leaving is typical for these sought after and limited camera beds that so many doctors vie for in scheduling their patients.

By now I know the drill, and should, considering the multiple times I've been hospitalized for this same test. Though boring and long, there is no pain or surgery involved. Given that my new neurologist really wants me to have it administered and evaluated at his facility—and that I trust him—encourages me to comply.

Once attached to the electrodes, monitoring proceeds similarly to that which I've had in the past. The big difference, however, is in the interpretation. Unlike former physicians overseeing it, his team recognizes it isn't that I'm not having seizures—but they are too quick to register on the monitors, (with only some inconclusive irregularities detected). Fortunately, abnormal jerking and other movements are visualized on camera, enabling the neurologist to come up with the most effective "cocktail" of medications for my specific symptoms. As a result, from this particular study forward, I have never appreciated such effective seizure control.

I think it is important to note that not only do patients remember negative doctor/patient encounters, but positive as well. Though my experience with the physician who emotionally shut the door on me, leaving me feeling ridiculed, demeaned, unheard and rushed—(but, most of all, in intense pain)—remains imbedded in my mind, I will never forget this specialist who restored my faith in neurologists by opening his door to me—at a time I needed him, (and to be heard)—most.

Subsequent to the hospitalization, and in compliance with my doctor's request, I busy myself looking for a nearby hospital with a 3.0 MRI scanner—one that is twice the strength of those I've used in the past and only a keypad away in locating—thanks to modern technology. Calling the nearest qualifying facility, I'm taken by surprise, in a positive way my exhilarated voice doesn't even pretend to hide, to learn they have an opening for this well-sought-after scanning machine for tomorrow—a Saturday morning, no less.

While being positioned on the conveyor-belt–like table, I ask the technician if I should expect to notice any difference in the length of time and/or noise as opposed to the past MRI scanning machines involving less intensity. Her answer is NOT what I expect—that the duration of this one will actually be shorter, with the volume approximately the same. There is something to be said for advances in technology! True to her word—and many silent prayers later that the scan will be meaningful—we leave within the half hour. When the results come back with multiple white spots on my brain stem, discernable due to visualization of an area not seen as precisely in the past, (because of lesser magnification), I am once again impressed by the competency of the physician who took that into consideration when ordering the stronger scan. While there is no "fix" for what occurred—to reflect these results—we now know the area effected and what symptomatic treatment may be appropriate, which is a lot better than where I was prior to switching to him.

CHAPTER NINE

Bragging Rights

"A Grandmother thinks of her grandchildren day and night, even when they are not with her. She will always love them more than anyone would understand."

—Karen Gibbs, A Gallery of Scrapbook Creations

Though I'm accustomed to the waves of excitement that ripple through my stomach—like a cascading waterfall—whenever we reach the last highway stop as we near the end of our four-plus hour drive to the home of one set of our grandchildren, they are particularly prevalent today. I'm reading in the classrooms of our two oldest grandsons—and I can't wait! While one may consider living a long distance away a disadvantage, I get the distinct sense the children don't feel in the least bit neglected as a result—most likely because of our determination to spend quality time with them on a very regular basis, (while keeping in touch by phone and computer communication in-between). By doing so, I feel such a part of their worlds. I know their individual strengths, likes and dislikes, friends' and teachers' names, favorite colors, games, activities they participate in, and so forth. It warms my heart that when something positive, (or even negative), occurs in their peer interactions, they feel confident in picking up the phone and calling to tell me all about it. This grandmother has celebrated sporting accomplishments and soothed injuries—long distance—with carefully chosen words of love. Hours have been spent concentrating on the things that are important to them at various stages of their lives. Whether it is what to do about having to sit next to a well-known bully, how to help disabled peers, critiquing a school newspaper one grandson initiated and authors on his own, (hmm, maybe genetics at play?), helping one who just learned they are getting the "meanest" teacher in the school next year and so forth, grandmothers are there to fulfill a role in their lives no one else can. I can still remember the patient and wise way my grandmother seemed to know just what to say, and how to say it—actually the very words she used, more than six decades ago—to make my world so special.

Even before ink transforms these to-date unspoken thoughts—cherished in the privacy of my mind—into typed words I never would have predicted I'd share with the world, (or at least that small part of it reading this book), my eyes bulge with about-to-overflow tears as warm memories of the moments I spent with my grandmother—Nonna—continue to inundate my head. Like a direct line from that reserved area of my heart, (the one only experiences with her occupy), memories of those unforgettably special times surface as clearly as if they happened yesterday. With a warm and reminiscent feeling overtaking me from head-to-toe, I think to myself how fortunate my grandchildren would be—if only I could be half the grandmother Nonna was!

To be honest, I'm not quite sure how my eldest grandson is going to handle the portion of my school visit where a student introduces his guest reader. Though undoubtedly secure enough to stand up before his class and present someone, what I wonder about is whether he will introduce me as his grandmother or by the special, inarguably unusual name I'm actually called. With an unmistakably proud smile across his face—confidence exuding from his voice—any question I had, no longer is, as my fourth grader announces, "All the way from Connecticut to read to us, this is Pa-Pa. Do you want to know how she got her name?". At this point he captures not only the curiosity of his classmates but his teacher, as well. He proceeds to explain that when he was less than a year old his parents excitedly told him Pa-Pa was coming to visit, and he somehow associated that as meaning both his grandmother and grandfather. To avoid the confusion of calling two people by the same name, especially as he got a few months older, his grandfather was re-named: Pa-Pa Ed—(which is sentimental to me given that our children called my dad Pa-Pa Red)—while I remained "Pa-Pa". Needless to say, it generates lots of enthusiastic discussion among the students, many of whom sharing that they, too, have "Pa-Pa's".

After a fleeting but enjoyable storytelling hour, and distribution of pre-approved, school-sanctioned snacks that correlated with the books I read, it is time to leave. Handing the teacher a book I purchased for donation to their classroom, the children are busied selecting the color snack they want—all except one. Bittersweet chills infiltrate my body when a little boy comes up and hugs me as he says, "I wish I had a Pa-Pa like you". Impulsively, and with no consideration as to whether the school would approve, I respond by hugging him back—a need I sense from him and am not about to ignore. My grandson later shares that this particular friend recently experienced a loss in his life. At that very moment, I silently vow to be his adoptive "Pa-Pa", giving him extra attention whenever I see him with my grandson.

Moving on to my younger grandson's classroom, it is with a different selection of age-appropriate books I intend to read to what I hope results in an equally attentive audience. The pride in his eyes as his friends vie for positions sitting close to me—while confident the coveted seat directly beside me is reserved for the person bringing the guest reader—is unmistakable. By now depleted-energy-challenged, it is beyond question that the love this little boy has in his heart for me, which is not only written all over his adoring face as his eyes look up into mine—but expressed in the way he tenderly strokes my arm sitting next to me as I read—is inarguably responsible for my transferring questionably possible intentions from my "I want to do this" brain cells—to determination activating my "I'm GOING to do this" cells.

Exhausted as I sink into the comfort of my daughter's car two hours after arriving at the elementary school, it is a good fatigue— knowing the afternoon was a success. Momentarily closing my eyes, I feel my face shape into a smile as I silently ask a question I can't answer, (or maybe I can!)—who had more fun, me or the children?

Fast-forward several years:

It is almost impossible to believe, as I sit here typing, that so many years have passed since four grandparents-to-be sat in the labor/delivery waiting room excitedly expecting their very first grandchild. How could I possibly now have a grandson who is old enough to work as a lifeguard—much less satisfy the age requirement to apply for a prerequisite learner's permit, with the intention of subsequently qualifying for a driver's license? No longer a child, he is now a grown young man—and what a thoughtful, mature one he turned out to be. I honestly don't know anyone his age who is more compassionate and loving toward others. I am so impressed with the way he is open-mindedly considerate to ALL his peers, unaffected by their popularity or what others think of them. Looking at his birthday invitation list was a real eye-opener for me. Sensitive to the feelings of others, he included classmates representing various social levels, some of whom rarely, (if ever), are asked to attend such events—which my grandson found unconscionable. He also reaches out to the disabled, doing all he can to assist and make their lives easier. Knowing classmates are hospitalized, especially for extended periods of time, he is the first to be there visiting them. He is patient with his younger sister's friends, even acquiescing when they ask him to read stories. I suspect he will choose a profession in which he works with disabled or disadvantaged individuals, as I see so much potential there. However, regardless of what field he selects, I have no doubt he will be a success.

Okay, I admit it, I am thrilled with my second grandson's writing ability. Not only is it creative and humorous, but appreciated by both his peers and teachers. Having demonstrated the initiative to request authoring a school newspaper—which was granted—he has written several issues to-date. Each was well- received, appropriate and pertinent to current topics of interest about his school and students his age. While inarguably accomplished in many areas, from sports to scholastics—which I commend seeing him pursue—my dream is that someday he will also write books. A talent like his deserves to be shared.

Although their youngest brother clearly aspires to be just like his big brothers, something commonly seen in families with older siblings, in truth, he needn't. He possesses so many remarkable attributes that belong just to him. Caring and easy going, always willing to help, agreeable—he is the student every teacher wants in their class. Versatile as he is, he gets along with all ages, a strength in his household considering the different age groups—and that of their frequently visiting friends. A natural athlete, he especially excels in running. As I look at his impish face with its broad smile, that immediately warms anyone's heart, I'm catapulted back in time—and just for one fleeting moment, as my mind plays tricks on me, (in a lovingly reminiscent way), it is the 1950's and I'm staring at my brother Al rather than my grandson. Sorting through pictures of my sibling at the same age corroborates the image my memory resurrects. They could be twins—and if they share not only physical—but personality characteristics as well, which I suspect they do—my grandson will mature to adulthood as a giving, generous, well-liked, great guy, too.

Okay, so cut me a little slack here—I only have one granddaughter. Truthfully, I'm not quite sure where to start—except to say she is multi-talented in a nice way. (Do I sound a little biased already?) Though she has had to step up to the plate, living in a family with three older brothers, she also is perceptive in recognizing them as some of her best protectors. She and I have had some thought-provoking talks about the advantages of being the only girl, (something I don't think she will fully appreciate until she is older)—at least I didn't. Like her, I envied my friends who had sisters to go home to and share "girl talk" with, play dress up, have tea parties, etc. It wasn't until I became an adult that I realized, firsthand, that brothers offer a perspective and friendship like none other—one I wouldn't trade for the world—which, I have no doubt, nor will she.

Currently pre-occupied with far less intense, life's experience adult reflection—and more immediate and age-appropriate thoughts—(which, though we can't see, know by the happiness she exudes on a daily basis, must result—at her level—in smiley faces multiplying daily throughout her mind)—she is immersed in the fun and carefree life all children deserve. From singing, to dancing, to combining both in parts she has been chosen for, she is loving life. Observing some of her behavior, at times she reminds me of her Aunt Storey at her age—probably because she is incessantly singing: when her parents are driving, when she is taking a bath, when she is in bed, etc. Though, like with Storey, the unrelenting melodies can—and at times do—drive her siblings up a wall, to me it is a refreshing indication of a very happy child. What more could parents, (and grandparents!), ask for?

When dropped off at school she literally bounds out of the car, into the welcoming company of friends awaiting her arrival. She loves learning and is an avid reader. Seeing her interact with her "Pa-Pa Ed" is like being in a time warp, watching him when our girls were her age. (Hmm, I wonder how tight someone can be wrapped around another's finger before the circulation is challenged—better keep an eye on it!) Her face lights up the moment she sees him. Together they practice her golf swings, basketball shots, softball pitching and anything that involves quality time together. Inarguably, his only granddaughter holds a special place in his heart—and she knows it! Fortunately, he has a big heart with LOTS of room for each of his grandsons, as well.

To summarize her qualities—not that I could ever fully do justice to all of them—what warms my heart most is that beside the typical things one would expect someone her age to demonstrate, (participation in arts and crafts, sports, sleep-overs, etc.), more importantly it is the caring person she is that stands out. Considerate to all, it comes as no surprise that she lives a life surrounded by friends and, most likely, always will.

Fast-forward even a few more years and I am now the "Pa-Pa" of six. Our daughter Storey and son-in-law Ravi's preschooler invited us to Thanksgiving dinner at his school and we can't wait to attend. Every classroom has been assigned preparation of one side dish to accompany the turkeys provided by the school staff. Walking noticeably faster than usual, as though he can't get there quick enough, to say our grandson is excited would be an understatement! Dressed in pilgrim attire the children made themselves, he holds my hand tightly, tugging on it gently—as if to direct me to where we need to go as we walk to his school. Despite his well-intentioned efforts, it is more accurately the enticingly mouth-watering aromas that escape the building, infiltrating our nostrils invitingly, that navigate us to the school's location—long before we enter it.

Proudly escorting us to our pre-assigned seats, he serves many of the courses, (in a much more grown-up way than I'm ready to see him fulfill). The smile overtaking his entire face tells me that while I may not be ready, he sure is! Contentedly stuffed, we leave his school having made a lifetime memory—does it get any better than that?

They may be the youngest but certainly not left out! At the time of this writing, the "little boy" described at the Thanksgiving pre-school dinner is now a big seven and his younger brother is almost four. Our seven-year-old is into swimming, soccer, chess, board games, math, various cultural opportunities, birthday parties, socializing with friends and many other age-appropriate activities. He is scholarly in nature with many future aspirations, any of which he could successfully pursue. He and I enjoy coin collecting together, an activity which, in addition to the hobby, is conducive to one-on-one uninterrupted conversations that are mutually appreciated.

A special memory I have of him occurred when he was about five. He gave me the biggest and best grandma smile, (oops, I mean "Pa-Pa" smile), I've ever received from a grandchild. It was during a memorial Mass that was being offered for "Grammy"—one his cousins were also attending—and he LOVES his cousins, (whom he hadn't seen in months). When he walked into the crowded, dimly-lit church, I followed his eyes as he methodically searched for them—noting the transformation from serious to elated, with an unmistakable sparkle lighting them up the minute he spotted them. Making a beeline for their pew, (unaware that we were in the one behind them, as his conscientious scrutiny ended the moment he discovered his cousins), it wasn't until halfway through the service that he happened to turn around and noticed me for the first time. I will never forget the ear-to-ear smile that reflected back at me from a surprised little boy who, upon initial recognition, touched his cheek to my hand—both of which were at about the same height—and warmed not only my hand, but my heart—forever.

At almost four, and my youngest, it is difficult to describe this grandson's interests in the same way I did the others because he is just beginning to express them. What I DO know is that he is into subways—evidenced by the fact that he can name them all, purchases toy renditions of the authentic ones any time he can, (trust me, they're not fun to step bare-footed on!), and expects me to identify them by number as easily as he can. He has an endearing personality and is a real joy to be around. Recently, we shared a special one-on-one day with him when he was off from school and his brother was not. Okay, so maybe we spoiled him JUST a little, (did I mention anything about a toy store, pizza, jumping-over-sidewalk-cracks game, selecting roses on his own to bring home to Mommy and going to a frozen yogurt shop with zillions of toppings—most of which he wanted and got?)—but it was such fun. The pride in his eyes when he handed Storey the flowers he "picked out all by myself"—and the smile that got bigger and bigger when she asked "Did you get these for ME?", as he enthusiastically nodded his head up and down, while snuggled into her arms as she lovingly hugged him, is a vision never to be forgotten in grandmothers' memory banks—at least not this one's!

One thing he especially enjoys when visiting us is the park conveniently located within walking distance, about a quarter of a mile away, on the street next to ours. It is designed particularly for younger children, with water sprays, heavy-duty plastic bucket-like swings, short slides and age-appropriate climbing apparatus—while at the same time offering equipment appealing to his older brother. On a good weather day, it is a win/win opportunity at Pa- Pa and Pa-Pa Ed's.

This Summer was particularly enjoyable because not only did we get to vacation with our entire family at the beach, including a few of my brothers and their families, but our granddaughter and niece, just months apart in age, had uninterrupted quality time—a treat they seldom get living four hours apart. It was like one long sleepover for both of them, not to mention having a friend to play with at the shore every day. A particularly heart-warming incident, which I look forward to describing to him when he is older, occurred when our youngest grandson decided he wanted to play soccer in the huge yard at the beach house—with the older kids. When unable to get the ball—which was most of the time—he would go out to the sidelines, select an out-of-play ball and start kicking it—regardless of the direction. Enablers that we are, the entire deck full of adoring relatives would clap and encourage him to do it more. Needless to say, the smile on his face for success he alone recognized in himself, was precious! Yes, being a grandmother, (or Pa-Pa, depending who you are talking to), is a blessing beyond description—and as much as authoring a book inarguably allows the opportunity to transfer those sentiments into words, all the ink on earth couldn't possibly replicate what it is really like!

Chapter Ten

Please God, Not My Husband!

"If you live to be a hundred, I want to live to be a hundred minus one day so I never have to live without you."

—Joan Powers, Pooh's Little Instruction Book.

"Hey, hon, can you take a look at this bump on my back and let me know what you think?", Eddie nonchalantly asks as he steps out of the shower. With the tone of his voice indicative of nothing serious, I automatically assume he has a bruise of some sort. Not seeing anything obvious, I run my hand over the lower left section of his back that he is pointing to. As I do, a cold chill makes my skin chicken-like bumpy at the realization that this is no bruise. What I feel is a golf ball sized lump under his skin—and it needs evaluation—NOW!

"I think it makes sense to show it to your primary care physician and get her opinion", I say as casually as possible, so as not to share my alarm with him, "after all, she's far more familiar with these things than I am". Whether denial—one of the emotions most of us initially turn to when a sudden, unexplained and potentially scary medical anomaly surfaces, temporarily kicked in— I can't say. I suspect, however, that my advice just confirmed what he was already thinking himself. Contacting his physician's office, we feel fortunate that a slot in her busy schedule is available just a few days from now.

Upon palpitation, her advice is that he should see a surgeon for a consultation. Unfortunately, the wait is much longer to see her, a few nerve-wracking months, to be exact. When the appointment finally arrives, the surgeon orders a needle biopsy scheduled for a week later. Because the results show lymph cells, a follow-up procedure to remove the entire mass is required, which she has an opening for in two weeks.

Praying silently in the waiting room of the hospital, it occurs to me that Eddie is either putting up a very good front or he is as nervous as I am, way down deep in his heart, where no one can see and only he can feel. If not, he is in big time denial. I want to take him in my arms and say it will be okay, but do I really know that? At the same time, I need someone to hold me in their arms and reassure me, but until I know his biopsy results, no one can— and will they be able to then?

Holding a full cup of by-now lukewarm coffee, one that seems tasteless because my mind and prayers can't concentrate on anything else but him, my hand shakes as I journal these thoughts. Optimistically expecting the surgical procedure to go well, it is the results that I am most concerned about. Reality is really hitting home today. Prior to his procedure, as he slept on the gurney, I reflected on how—as much as we don't necessarily want to get older, or feel that we are, it is happening right before our very eyes—quicker than we ever could have imagined. Ironically, it is not the number we find difficult, but the deteriorating health that all-too-often accompanies that escalating age. Realistically, are any of us ever prepared for that, much as we know it happens? Yes, we may have seen illness in older relatives or in friends our own ages, but it is far different when it is your best friend, specifically the spouse who has been your major confidant throughout your marriage. Dear God, please let him be okay. The quiet eeriness of the hospital waiting room unnerves me. Other than recipes repeatedly described on a cooking show which I'm totally disinterested in at the moment, the silence is deafening. Besides, who can concentrate on food when my husband is undergoing removal of a potentially serious mass?

Tick tock, tick tock, the metronome inside my head drones on far too slowly for me. Minutes seem like hours as five minutes into Eddie's surgery I feel like we've been here all day, and even more frustratingly, it will take up to two weeks, post-surgery, for the pathology results—two long weeks, I'm sure. Until then, we will be on pins-and-needles knowing nothing.

My thoughts are interrupted by an assumption regarding another family, one that isn't difficult to make. While in the waiting room, doctors and nurses have updated patients' families publicly, within earshot of strangers they never met. Consequently, when a nurse enters the waiting room and asks a couple to come into a private room to talk, I immediately think this means trouble. It resurrects a memory in a sad chamber of my heart, the same type of little room that a physician took our family into when he broke the news to us that my ears didn't want to hear—that my dad's death was imminent. Had I been a child, I probably would have done what I remember children doing when I was small, (myself included)—blocked my ears with my hands, making anatomical ear muffs as I yelled, "I can't hear you". Tempted as I was, adult maturity taught me how futile this effort was. Oh, if only life's challenges could be rectified so easily!

As the door of the little conference room opens, I'm taken by surprise—in a good way—when I see the faces of the couple, (who only minutes before followed the nurse in), transformed from consternation to relief. Much like a student anxious about his test score as his teacher is distributing graded exams, others can "read" how they did by the expression on his face the moment he sees it— and trust me, this couple is pleased with their "score"! Overhearing their discussion regarding where they want to go to lunch as they gather their belongings and leave the facility, my conscience gently cautions me not to jump to conclusions which often result in misjudgments because they are not always accurate—which, in this case, they fortunately were not.

Within what seems like days, but is only an hour, Eddie's procedure is over and I'm allowed to sit with him in recovery. Multi-tasking during this time, not only do I visit with him but I also get a lesson from his nurse learning how I'm to apply the dressing. Once he has been sufficiently monitored—which amounted to about two hours—we are on our way home. While he feels fine and exhibits no repercussions from the surgery, waiting for results is a much more anxiety-inducing challenge.

"You DO have an oncologist, don't you?" this surgeon I've only met once asks in a cavalier, expectant voice implying doesn't everyone—and, if not, we are negligent. No! This CAN'T be the way we're going to learn my husband has cancer, with the most uncompassionate, insensitive delivery possible. Imagining my blood boiling, I can feel the warm flush of my face which, though unable to visualize it at the moment, is no doubt coloring at the speed of an express elevator—rising from the bottom floor to the top with no stops in between. Angry beyond words, it takes all the restraint I can manage not to retaliate with, "Sure, you idiot, his name and phone number are on a magnet on our refrigerator, right next to that of our family dentist. After all, doesn't EVERYONE have an oncologist?"

Instead, with unmistakable and well-deserved attitude, I respond to her question with, "Why? Does he need one?" Not only does her answer come across as demeaning and insensitive, but it gives the impression that we are ignorant for not having an oncologist—which doesn't make sense considering we've received no results yet—and she is aware that is the purpose of this appointment. Consequently, we are momentarily stunned silent when, looking at her chart instead of us, she responds, "Of course he does—he has Non-Hodgkin's Type B Lymphoma". Recovering enough to let my logical thinking replace the emotional, I take Eddie's hand, look into understandably shocked and impossible-to- hide scared eyes and say with conviction I pray I can fulfill, "We WILL get through this—TOGETHER". With the doctor abruptly leaving the room to call an oncologist, we take advantage of the privacy—not only to share some quiet time attempting to process what we've just learned—but to call our daughters to discuss the results, (which we promised we would do as soon as we got them).

Stacey's nurse practitioner background automatically kicks in. Having researched his symptoms and accurately predicted his diagnosis weeks earlier, she is immediately clinically reassuring, reminding us that it is one of the most curable cancers, especially caught at such an early stage. (Later, she admits part of the optimism she verbalized was for our benefit—and that she had to take several deep breaths before calling us back.)

Storey, on the other hand, reacts to the results in a more emotional way. "Mom, you sound like you need a hug, (She's right about that!), I'm sorry I'm not there to give you one". "Me too, hon", my voice croaks out, cracking midway despite my concerted effort to keep it from doing so. My heartstrings tug when her next words ask, "May I talk to dad?", because I know what is coming. Handing him the phone, he immediately reassures her, "Sto, I'm going to be fine. This is just a little bump in the road". Listening, I can't help but think he is sugar-coating his words for the benefit of both of us, neither of whom is buying them at the moment. Looking at me while still talking to her, he wordlessly runs a finger down each of his cheeks to convey to me that she is crying, a visual gesture that makes my eyes fill and my heart ache.

To daughters, a father can be their world. I know my dad was to me and still is, in the priceless memories I hold in a special part of my heart reserved just for him. It is a place I still go to, silently, for advice, comfort, etc.—a location only he and I can, and always will, share. On my bedroom wall is a picture of him playing with me on my blanket on the floor when I was about five months old. He looks so proud and, even at that young age, I'm looking up into his eyes adoringly. Under the picture, I hung an anonymous saying I found, "DAD—A SON'S FIRST HERO, A DAUGHTER'S FIRST LOVE". How true! Having experienced the father/daughter bond, firsthand, it is re-ignited in me as I observe it in our adult daughters. Though Stacey and Storey demonstrate it in different ways, each of their relationships are so very powerful—and it is especially at times like this I thank God that they are.

Leaving the surgeon's office, we take advantage of advice Storey had given me on the phone—to do something fun. Actually, even before her recommendation, suspecting the results might not be what we were hoping for, we selected a movie at a local theater that we have been wanting to see, the intent being to distract ourselves in a positive way, followed by dinner at a restaurant we often frequent—a place where especially today our innermost thoughts would understandably surface—in the comfort of the familiar, while at the same time the topic couldn't be more foreign to us.

Before going to the theater, Eddie stops to get a soft drink as we have some time to kill—and he is undoubtedly dry from trying to process the heavy information he was just given. Taking advantage of the privacy this affords, I call a few of my brothers. Reaching my brother Al, our conversation seems surreal. Normally a very private person, as I share Eddie's diagnosis I'm crying my eyes out standing in front of a coffee shop where a bus full of people unload, wiggling in line, shifting from foot-to-foot, undoubtedly exercising all the control they can muster, waiting as patiently as possible for their turns to use the limited-stall bathrooms. Despite also anxious for their cups of joe, let's face it, priorities are priorities!

It is like our news just registered as I relate the diagnosis to my sibling, almost unaware anyone else is here—at least not in my world. Oblivious as I am to these strangers, suddenly they are all approaching me with arms I've never felt before hugging me in comfort, telling me everything will be all right. How do they know? They don't even know what's wrong. What they do know and demonstrate, however, is heartfelt compassion. I can see it in eyes that have never met mine before and feel it as they transfer it to me—and, in a way I can't explain, it makes me feel better.

As these kind strangers go into the coffee shop, I remain outside experiencing an awkward moment, almost like when someone inappropriately laughs nervously at a funeral. Describing to my brother that I am laughing and crying at the same time, in front of people I don't know, (which should embarrass me but doesn't), the unlikely scenario I depict gets him going, too. The entire experience proves cathartic in that my spirits are lifted when Eddie returns only minutes later, allowing me to be the positive support I need and want to be for him.

Overwhelmed with conflicting and powerful emotions my brain cells aren't prepared to fully process, it is almost ironic that while watching the movie, THE INTERN, one of the stars advises a younger intern to always be prepared with a handkerchief in the event that the woman he is with needs one. During a very poignant moment, as I try to register the diagnosis Eddie was just given, one I wish was just a bad dream we will wake up from, (but know, deep down inside, isn't), Eddie reaches into his pocket and hands me a tissue—and, once again, by this sensitive and intuitive gesture—I'm reminded, for the umpteenth time, why I fell in love with this man.

Eddie's doctor, the oncologist he has yet to meet, called him at work today. I know he appreciated the support and compassion the call demonstrated, especially in contrast to the negative experience with his previous physician. By answering as many questions as he could, without the benefit of scan results, he provided a sense of security at a very unsettling time.

Explaining that he arranged for a P.E.T. scan on the same day of his first appointment, but a few hours prior so that he could have the results when we come in, it is obvious that his treatment began with the phone call rather than his first visit.

If eyes could type, the words, "I am so fortunate to have this doctor I haven't even met yet", reflect back at my inquiring ones when Eddie walks into the house that night. Relief relaxes his face, removing lines that seem to have disappeared for the first time since he heard the diagnosis. He is obviously impressed with this physician already—and so am I!

Even though his appointment is only a week away it seems like an eternity, leaving us feeling somewhat like little children who love school waiting for the last few days of summer vacation to end. The difference is that unlike the analogy of the excitedly anxious children, our reasons for the anticipated day to get here are far more critical, and potentially life-changing.

Prior to a preliminary x-ray, the technician informs me that though I will understandably not be allowed in the room during Eddie's picture-taking due to radiation exposure, I am certainly welcome during his P.E.T. scan.

Because the machine is so loud and Eddie is partially obscured by the donut-like equipment, he is unaware that I am even there, which isn't the important thing—it's that I am. Besides, the technician informs him that I just came in. Sitting and listening to the noisy, rhythmic hum of the machine, nowhere near as loud as an M.R.I. but impossible to miss all the same, I'm suddenly struck by how all alone in their own physically challenged world patients are. Despite the fact that I'm in the room at this moment, the machine owns him. Just for now, he belongs more to "it" than me. Though I want to be on the table with him, reassuring everything will be all right, holding his hand in mine, I can't. He says nothing, lying perfectly still as instructed, while various colors of light, one at a time, pass over him. Watching from my chair, approximately two car lengths beyond his feet, I'm barely aware of its uncomfortable steel back, too consumed praying that this full body scan reveals no additional cancer.

Interrupting my prayers comes a memory of a sentiment I heard way back when, that seeing a rainbow is a positive sign. On the way to the hospital a few hours ago, Eddie spotted one in the distance and, as we were walking into the clinic Stacey called from her out-of-state home to share that she saw two this morning. I'll happily go with that!

Time to stop writing and read the Holy Water reflections I brought to the scan. My cousin—who went to Lourdes—shared those and some of the water he brought back from there with us, which we blessed ourselves with prior to leaving the house this morning. Known for its healing properties, it is something I believe strongly in.

Whether it is apprehension on my part or a mix-up in scheduling I cannot say, but this scan seems to be taking forever. We were told forty-five minutes and we've been here at least twice that long. What could THAT indicate? I don't even want to go there!

Finally, the technicians slide Eddie out from under the machine and I get my first glimpse of him since coming into the cold, sterile room. To me, he looks pale, innocent and scared, which he undoubtedly is. As much as he refers to his health condition as just a "bump in the road", his blood pressure is elevated and he has had a nervous stomach. Maybe denial is an effective coping mechanism for him, (or is it?), but I'm not buying his brave front—convinced his well-intentioned efforts are for the benefit of me and our daughters. As someone who has known and loved him for so long, I see right through it.

Initially getting to know him as the girl who lived across the street, I shared giddy, flirtatious daily phone calls with him—talks and advice about each other's dates, college course selections, best picks for professors, etc. I saw him graduate from college, while he was solely responsible for me doing so, as well. Before my then co-ed eyes, he transformed from a teenager to a man, one who has proven to be the best husband, father, grandfather, son-in-law, brother, brother-in-law, friend, etc. anyone could ask for—and then some!

Every month of our now forty-five-year marriage, he celebrated our "month-a-versary", (as he labeled them when he started the tradition a month after our wedding). Please, God, let him continue this touching way of commemorating our special day for many, many years. Allow Stacey's idol, the person she refers to as "the smartest man in the world", continue to prove to her that he is, in countless ways, for a long, long time to come. Allow our family to go on referring to Storey as "Daddy's little deodorant stick", a name she acquired due to pictures of her, every year of her childhood, with her head in the crook of his arm—the safest, most secure place she knew.

Unable to stop my trip down memory lane, as the technician hands Eddie his clothes my mind reverts back to a time when personal computers were virtually non-existent in private homes— and we were one of very few families to own one. Since Eddie's profession is Informational Technology, computers are his specialty—an area he has been proficient in for decades. One year when Stacey was in elementary school, he created a cartoon birthday invitation using characters on the keyboard to print out the shape of an animal, inviting her friends to a unique computer party. Taking the day off from work, he taught the children who attended basic computer skills, along with take-homes of their new-found knowledge. To say it was an innovative hit would be an understatement!

Perhaps a memory that to this day touches me most was his dedication to coaching. It wasn't just the fact that as a father he made himself available for both girls' softball ball teams, but what he had to do to make it happen. In our town, after coaching a team for several years, if the position was relinquished, it was understandably given to someone else. Because Storey had to wait a year after Stacey became too old to play—before making the age requirement for softball—Eddie secured the position of coaching his youngest daughter, as well, by continuing to coach the team during that interim year when he had no daughters of his own on it. Now if that isn't dad commitment, I don't know what is!

"Stop it!", the few logical brain cells that remain active at the moment silently scream to the illogical ones that currently appear to outnumber them. Remember what multiple medical professionals have told us: This is NOT a death sentence! Besides, with Eddie dressed and ready following his scan, I now have more important things to concentrate on.

Doing my best to curve my lips into the most believable smile, (unfortunately, not to me), I give him a hug and we head to lunch prior to his initial early afternoon oncology appointment.

Entering the hospital following an all-too-brief meal—one I

wanted to go on forever—I once again beg the magical thinking part of my brain to convince me this is nothing more than a bad dream—but undeniable reality kicks in as I'm overwhelmed by an emotion that engulfs me to the depths of my soul—FEAR.

It is already unlike any facility neither he, nor I, have been to. Beginning with the fact that it is a cancer center, according to every sign associated with it—from the parking garage, to the elevators, down the hallways and into the reception area—there is nothing left to speculation as to why a patient comes here. Every sign I read is a disturbing reminder of the gravity of Eddie's situation—making me scared for him, (and me!).

The dedication of every staff member to go out of their way, to be kind and accommodating, is incredible. From housekeepers, to coffee shop employees, to scrub-donned medical staff passing us in the hallways, you name it—it's like being engulfed in a group hug by a well-trained staff who, through experience has come to recognize the scared, chalky white, disoriented faces of those who need it most.

Though my lips somehow respond to their courteousness as politely as I can, anything I say and do at this point is involuntary. Actually, I feel a little like I did post-brain stem stroke. People are talking to me in a surreal world where I don't even register half of what they are saying. For me, they fade in and out, kind of like clouds when you are in an airplane. As in that situation, there are times you pass through them oblivious of their presence. Though my body is obviously not capable of passing through people, it is like my mind, in its own way, is protecting the clutter of extraneous distraction, allowing me to concentrate on expectations regarding the only person I'm interested in meeting at the time—Eddie's oncologist.

With my thoughts consumed by horrific memories of how coldly his biopsy results were delivered, I'm starting to fear that all doctors practicing in specialties with the potential of delivering undesirable and/or life-threatening results are trained to erect a callous and impossible-to-penetrate wall between themselves and their patients—possibly for their own protection. After all, if they became too emotionally involved, would they still be effective in a profession where dispensing unfavorable results are sometimes a reality they are responsible for? From my firsthand perspective, I advocate that doctors take the risk of showing their human side. Patients gravitate toward physicians who are brave enough to do so—at least I do!

Looking at Eddie, not knowing what lies before him as we open the door to his doctor's reception area, he readily accepts my extended hand. Curling it around mine I say to him, in a subdued but reassuring voice only we can hear, the words I've been saying all along, "We'll get through this together". Lightly squeezing my fingers is his way of privately conveying that my support is appreciated, though I'm not sure at this point I'll be able to validate this assertion without convincing medical back up, which, to date, we don't have. Once again, I'm reminded of how alone the patient really is in fighting such challenging battles.

Having even more compassion than ever for others who have walked this journey, my goal is to leave his appointment far more reassured than we are now; At the same time, my realistic brain cells fight to be heard—accomplished doctors who go above and beyond trying everything at their disposal to treat patients with serious illness are still limited by the parameters of today's medical technology. Hopefully it will be advanced enough for Eddie's condition.

Any concerns regarding the oncologist we've been referred

to prove unwarranted when we are taken aback—in a good way—the moment he enters the exam room. With a warm, immediately put-one-at-ease smile, he introduces himself by his first and last name, omitting his title. By doing so, he refreshingly demonstrates that he is no "doctor god", which means he has already passed my test!

Extending a hand not only to Eddie, but to me as well, further impresses me. I interpret his perception and body language as an indication that he "gets it"—we are a team. I have no intention of accompanying Eddie to his visits only to sit in the exam room like an invisible, speechless presence. He is my spouse and best friend. My opinions and questions can, and WILL, count.

Reviewing Eddie's biopsy results with us, it becomes clear even to untrained medical minds that he has insufficient information to accurately diagnose at this point. What he does suspect, however, is the potential for one of two possibilities: either very aggressive treatment requiring strong chemotherapy for several days as an inpatient or mild, out-patient radiation of short duration. The unknown, which will determine treatment, is whether his cancer has spread. Complicating the decision is the fact that his shoulder unexpectedly lit up on the P.E.T. scan—in addition to his back, (the latter of which was no surprise subsequent to removal of the mass because it is impossible to get every cell). Considering Eddie hurt his shoulder during the past six months, the question now is whether it is his injury the doctor is observing on the scan—or cancer that has infiltrated another part of his body. Evidence that he is too good a specialist to leave it to chance is proven when he makes the decision to order an ultrasound to further define the shoulder inflammation, to which we all agree. Treatment will depend on the results.

Curiously, though patients have been known to wait a

week or more for an available ultrasound slot, Eddie's physician scheduled his for tomorrow. Almost able to visualize the red flag that unfurls—at least on the television screen of my mind—(like a folding rain umbrella when its Velcro strap is released, prior to pushing the button to fully extend it)—I will the silent yet powerful image only I can see to remain just that—an unnecessary warning stored in my, at the moment, understandably-overactive worry brain cells—one that never materializes into anything further. But the depiction is so real the chill it evokes sends chicken-skin-like goose bumps running up and down my back. For the first time, I'm aware that there is immediacy associated with one of his potential treatments—and his doctor isn't wasting any time!

On the way home from the ultrasound the following afternoon, Eddie's cell phone rings. Because he is at the wheel and it is illegal to talk with a hand held one while driving in our state, I answer it. Having just left the facility where the scan was done, I'm surprised to hear it is his doctor—with results! Talk about efficiency, we haven't been on the road more than a half hour.

Involuntarily holding my breath, my body's way of attempting to brace itself in preparation for results I may not be ready to hear, I release a loud sigh, the volume of which only stored excessive air could make—(and, at any other time would embarrass me)—as the oncologist describes a significant muscle tear identified in his shoulder, rather than cancer that has spread. Hearing this, I can actually feel the sides of my mouth curl into a smile I can't see, but know defines my entire face with relief.

Informing me with conviction I find convincing and reassuring, that mild, out-patient radiation is all that will be required, I motion the thumbs up to Eddie as the physician verbalizes what the treatment plan already reveals—the cancer remains localized to the lower, left back, which is the area we originally addressed. It is the injury to the shoulder that caused that portion of his scan to light up, which we'll take over the other alternative—any day! For the first time in weeks, I can feel myself relax, molding my body into the supple leather of the car's seat, leaving its temporary impression, as I tell the physician he made my day. With all the compassion of a doctor who knew we would be counting the seconds waiting for the phone to ring, he gently tells me that is why he called. My admiration and respect for this specialist grows with every encounter. Floating on a cloud we did not expect to ride—but gratefully accept—we optimistically await his much less invasive treatment than what could have been, to begin.

For some, winning the lottery would be one of their biggest dreams come true. They fantasize ahead, almost incessantly, as to what they would do with the money. To me, we've just "won" something FAR more important—that no amount of money in the world even comes close to!

Today Eddie begins the first of his three and a half weeks of radiation. Stoically, he tells me I don't have to go with him. After all, each treatment only takes a few minutes and it isn't like I can go in the room with him. Excuse me, but is he insane? Does he think for one minute that I'm not going to be with him, as much as possible, through this entire journey? Were the words, "In sickness and in health" too long ago to remember? In truth, I know he is doing his best not to scare me, but who is there to wrap their arms around HIS bravely concealed fears and try to hug them away, if not me? Though like medical science I have my limitations, make no mistake when it comes to my husband I have every intention of stretching them to the fullest extent—and beyond!

After telling him I love him, (as if that was necessary!), I watch as he follows the technician down the inaccessible-to-me corridor leading to foreign and undoubtedly unnerving territory. Though he would disagree, from my perspective I look at him through eyes that no longer see the same person. Suddenly, he is vulnerable, fragile and dependent on treatments I'd prefer he didn't need to resort to. Excepting that we're adults, as I watch him disappear beyond my visual focus, I feel a little like a powerless mom watching her child led to the operating room, unable to accompany him—nor to influence the outcome—and my heart cries invisible tears.

Several prayers and cups of hot chocolate later, (with only one staff note instructing visitors how to CORRECTLY use the coffee machine—hmm, I wonder whose "flood" in the waiting/reception area initiated that!)—Eddie's treatments conclude. When they do, a two-month post-radiation period is initiated, which is the designated amount of time before re-scanning to determine if the treatment was effective. As discreetly as possible I find myself watching him at all times of the day—in various situations—and am relieved with what I observe. Unlike before treatment, he no longer comes home from golf requiring a three-hour nap due to intense fatigue, his color has improved from greyish white to pink and, in general, he appears much healthier—until the third week post-radiation, that is.

Walking into the living room and finding him in a deep sleep, with his head in his hand much like "the thinker", denial refuses to prevent me from resurrecting—from memory cells I'd hoped were destroyed—when he exhibited such intense fatigue before. Unfortunately, within minutes it becomes clear that these unwanted negative memory cells were never annihilated—in fact, far less compassionate than the out-numbered denial cells unsuccessfully trying to protect me, they appear to be winning.

Hoping this is just a fluke, it becomes disconcertingly obvious that it isn't when I witness a repeat scenario only two days later. Discouragingly, my mind can no longer even attempt to deny what my eyes can't miss—that deeper, sounder sleep that is atypical for him, midday—the intensity of which I can only remember him exhibiting a few times in our marriage—to be exact, just before starting radiation.

As he begins to stir only minutes later I do my best, despite nervous body language, (chills, hair standing straight up on my arms like quills of a porcupine, dry mouth, etc.), to conceal my innermost fears: that the lymphoma is back. At the same time, I need more information. In an effort to procure it, in the calmest, most matter-of-fact-voice I can execute, I ask, "Hon, how are you feeling"? "Fine", he replies. "Why, are you worried about me?" "No", I lie. "It just seems like you've been a little tired lately." A little? That's a stretch! Fortunately, before he can question my suspicions further, the telephone rings.

Walking into the oncologist's exam room I'm prepared—as prepared as one can be that is. Based on the changes I've observed in Eddie during the last two weeks, I'm not expecting the results of the P.E.T. scan to be normal. On the other hand, I'm not a doctor. Hopefully my untrained medical mind is in overdrive when it comes to evaluating him, and what I'm observing is nothing more than an anxious wife's exaggerated worst fears manifesting rather than the return of lymphoma.

Before time permits any further analytical thinking on my part, there is a knock on the door followed by the oncologist's entrance. Scrutinizing as I do, disappointingly I'm unable to interpret his poker straight eyes, meaning this impatient spouse has to wait for him to deliver the outcome of Eddie's test results.

Perceptively, he accurately demonstrates that he reads our fear and apprehension by getting right to the results, rather than prolonging our anxiety further. Pulling up his P.E.T. scan on the computer, he points to a miniscule area of inflammation found on a different area of his body, too small to locate upon palpitation—yet definitely indicative of close monitoring.

With the day of Eddie's repeat P.E.T. scan quickly approaching, I find myself intensifying my prayers—as the reassuring optimism that pulsated through my veins during initiation of the post radiation period no longer does. Discouraging pessimism now travels that same journey, uninvited. Much as I want to ignore and dismiss its presence, my silent intuition won't let me.

Not to overlook any potential complications at their earliest stages, an ultrasound of this recently uncovered area is scheduled for the following week. Understandably curious to hear those results as soon as possible, we give him permission to convey them to either of us and/or leave them on our voice mail. A chill of goose bumps prickles my spine with more fear than I've known to date, when he asks whether we want him to do so regardless of the news, good or bad. Without hesitation, we give him the okay, either way, but the question haunts me—in the office and even more lying in bed during the impenetrably quiet wee hours of the night, wondering what potentially bad news might be discovered. Annoyed with myself for even "going there" at such a preliminary stage, I turn to prayer that puts me at peace—and grants me sleep within minutes.

With the ring of Eddie's cell phone, I involuntarily hold my breath. Having just had his ultrasound, we are well aware that his physician wastes no time in reporting results—a characteristic we BOTH appreciate. If you think about it, regardless of when the diagnosis is delivered, it isn't going to change—so why not hear it at its earliest, most effectively treatable stage, my practical brain cells try to convince me—while my emotional ones run interference.

I can tell from the serious look of concentration on Eddie's face— forehead lines deeper and more prominent than usual, tight lips that show no evidence of a smile, etc., that I've guessed the caller correctly. If eyes could hear, the pensive look in his tells me he just learned something was found—and not in a good way. From what I can overhear, the defined area is once again miniscule—and in the same place that the other scan showed, which, on palpitation was too small to appreciate. Despite what some may interpret as encouraging signs, I still worry—with sweaty palms and a dry throat, in conjunction with skipped breaths—manifesting as physical giveaways that I can't conceal, even if I want to.

My hearing suddenly reacting as though it is on steroids, I block out all distractions—with ears selective only to Eddie's voice. The intensity of our topic makes me oblivious to the songs on the car's radio, nearby traffic, etc., clinging to his every word as he continues to reiterate what the doctor said. Filling in the holes of information I missed from the one-sided conversation I overheard, he explains that due to the positive results, rather than wait the six months as originally planned for re-scanning, it is scheduled for six weeks— again trying to determine if it could be a bruise or the spread of lymphoma. Knowing this physician never would have made this scheduling change if the results hadn't raised some red flags in his experienced mind, I have all I can do to hide my frustration. Six weeks? Why so long, the place in my brain no one can hear except me asks, silently? Before I have a chance to verbalize this concern in a way that doesn't come across as fearful to Eddie, he continues, explaining that amount of time is about how long it would take for a bruise to disappear—while a cancer could increase in size, further defining the diagnosis.

After six long, nerve-wracking weeks, that seemed far more like six years, the scans are repeated and the results come back— NEGATIVE, meaning that at the moment he is cancer-free. With a voice reflecting undisguised relief and satisfaction, his oncologist selects a larger gap between now and his next appointment. (Hmm, is there such a thing as the opposite of a red flag?) While cautioned to call him if we notice anything suspicious in the interim, he tells us he is optimistic that we won't. Does it get any better than that?

CHAPTER ELEVEN

Anaphylaxis 101

"When you get to the end of your rope,
tie the knot and hang on." —Franklin D.
Roosevelt

Mirrors are unkind to me as embarrassing bright pink, clown- like cheeks reflect their unnatural images back, similar to those of a little girl playing dress-up, having overdone her make-up. With a face that swells and colors more by the minute, my concern is undeniable—and I suspect legitimate.

After a six-month hiatus—a very painful six months—I resumed a biologic infusion drug two days ago and, at the moment, I feel like a child experiencing a sore throat with no clinical evidence of a fever, etc., unsuccessfully trying to convince a parent she shouldn't go to school. The raised, skeptical-appearing eyebrows of the physician at the Emergency Department, in conjunction with his laidback demeanor, (in contrast to one which might have initiated immediate treatment, indicating that this is time-sensitive), confirms that he gives little plausibility to my theory—that the itching I'm experiencing throughout my body is a reaction to the drug I was recently infused with. Trying to reassure me that had this been a reaction to the medication it would have occurred immediately after the infusion—not a day later—tells me I interpreted his body language accurately. (Hmm, no disrespect intended, but did you take Delayed Drug Reactions 101? my mind begs to ask but my voice refuses to utter.) Unconvinced with his assessment but in no apparent distress, I ingest the mild antihistamine he offers for my peace of mind and, when the itch begins to subside, I exit the medical facility.

Relieved that the doctor saw no reason for me to discontinue the infusions that have a positive effect on my autoimmune diseases, despite my concerns about a reaction, I optimistically choose to believe the next one won't cause a reaction.

Fast forward four weeks, it is disconcerting to realize—but impossible to deny—the incredible intensification of the unwanted symptoms' reappearance as the biologic begins to wear off and, the scary thing is, I'm not the only one to notice. Besides family and friends, strangers are quick to come to my assistance—observing disabilities I embarrassingly can no longer hide.

In restaurants, I'm unable to get up from a chair without self-consciously leaning most of my upper torso on the table top, using it for leverage as I push against it with my hands. The grunting and moaning this effort entails is involuntary—which, for a proud person, is the epitome of chagrin. My only consolation is that my next biologic infusion is in two weeks.

After two weeks that seemed far more like six, it is still dark, with bitterly colder-than-usual-temperatures, when my too-good-to-be-true friend, Denise, picks me up at 5:00 A.M. in order to catch our early train into the city. Other than Eddie,

Denise is the first person to accompany me to one of my infusions—though I'm thankful to say many have offered. How fortunate I am to have the supportive network I do!

Not surprisingly, with so much in common the longer than I'd like ride into the city doesn't lack for conversation. Before we realize it the inside of the train darkens, signaling our arrival at the underground tunnel section of the huge mass-transit station. Gathering our belongings, we exit the train onto the platform where we are immersed into the momentum of hundreds of commuters rushing toward their respective destinations. Willing myself to concentrate on leaving the platform area as quickly as possible—rather than watching how close to the edge of those deep drops to the tracks far-too-many passengers seem to come—the sunlit, architecturally impressive portion of the station, now within feet away, is a welcome sight.

Arriving well in advance of my appointment—and unaffected by the time constraints many commuters face rushing to work—we enjoy a delicious and relaxing breakfast. (Why can't they make bagels like this where we live?). When we are done eating, we hail a taxi that delivers us to the door of the infusion site. Loyally, Denise sits patiently across from me during the entire three-and-a-half-hour procedure, as potent but potentially symptom-altering chemicals infiltrate my veins, with the goal being better disease management and associated pain relief.

Chilled by the liquid that is stored under refrigeration and remains cold as it circulates throughout my body, like rivers of too-thin-to-skate-on ice, I gratefully accept the warm blanket the nurse provides. That, in addition to the fleece throw I brought from home, my Winter jacket and the medicine given in conjunction with the biologic—which makes me tired—send me guiltily off into sandman land, leaving Denise in the silent companionship of her crossword puzzle.

I'm momentarily disoriented as I awaken—until I see Denise's smile reflect back at me, which triggers my memory as to where we are and why. Dismissing my apologies for inadvertently leaving her without company for so long, the treatment ends. With the satisfaction of knowing that within a couple of days my pain will be significantly reduced, we are on our way.

Still tired, I sleep on the train most of the ride home—leaving Denise to singlehandedly challenge the computer in Scrabble. As she drops me off at my condo after what seems like only minutes— but in actuality is hours later—I say a silent prayer for a friend like her. Waking up the next day, I'm again reminded of her thoughtfulness, (as though I needed any MORE reminders!), when, while getting ready for our weekly coffee group—one that several of us have been regularly attending for more than thirty years—she calls and offers to swing by and give me a ride. Still a little weak from the infusion, this is a kindness I can't refuse.

By the time breakfast ends and I'm back home, exhaustion once again overcomes me. Curling up inside a snuggly warm fleece, like an unborn caterpillar in its cocoon, I'm asleep in the reclining chair within minutes. Awakening prematurely though still groggy, I think nothing of the itching in my right arm—until it continues to intensify after I scratch it. Inarguably superseding the need to satisfy my exhaustion, I cannot sleep nor ignore the incessant itching. Before long, my left arm feels mosquito-bite-infested as well. Recognizing this is most likely another reaction to the infusion, I once again head to a local medical facility. Fortunately, I live in an area where I have multiple choices within a comfortable driving distance. For the purpose of continuity, I select the one I went to after my last infusion. Though I don't sense immediate danger during the ride, there is no doubt in my mind that I am reacting more seriously and systemically than the first time. (As I write this

I can feel my body cringe thinking of what one of my best friends in the world—an experienced paramedic—would say about my driving myself. I don't even want to go there!). With a sigh of relief as the building comes into view, the silent, now guilt-ridden contemplation I find impossible to stop, whose message is difficult to dismiss even to myself—subsides. I know his concern would be justified—especially as I enter the facility unable to ignore the sensation of my throat tightening and hearing that is atypical for me—kind of like a hollow echo, similar to being underwater or traveling at a high altitude before one's ears pop.

When the registrant hears that I am here for a possible drug reaction, she tells me someone will be right out. Sitting in the surprisingly close-to-empty waiting room, a person dressed in purple scrubs appears within five minutes—understandably struggling with my last name—which isn't pronounced even close to the way it is spelled. Without an introduction, smile or anything that even comes close to resembling a warm and fuzzy, reassuring gesture, at a time I could use it most, I'm told, "Follow me", in a curt, unwelcoming voice.

As he takes my blood pressure, I struggle to see the identification badge attached to his belt—but his rotund physique and accompanying pot belly overlaps it, blocking it from my view. Not knowing his credentials, I decide to take a chance that he has a nursing degree and ask if he knows how long the drug I've taken stays in one's system. His abrupt and judgmental response takes me off-guard, as he looks me up and down and says, "In fat people it takes longer because it gets trapped in fat cells".

Before I have time to reflect on that cold and callous answer, (talk about the pot calling the kettle black!), or contemplate how someone with a personality such as his was able to successfully effectuate a job interview, without demonstrating the compassion and professionalism medical staff members really should possess, (unless he was more convincing to those considering him for the position than to this patient he is subsequently treating), a woman also dressed in scrubs walks in—her badge partially obscured at her waist. After about ten minutes of questioning, she concludes by informing me that she is going to order a large, one-time dose of steroids to be administered immediately. With a bewildered expression I can't see but feel transforming my face from confusion, as my eyes stretch open wider and my mouth drops agape, I ask "Who are you?" Her complexion coloring to crimson embarrassment, she awkwardly replies in a stuttered response that she is an A.P.R.N.—and because they are so busy she didn't get a chance to introduce herself. Within the hour, after ingesting the steroid and beginning to feel its positive effects, I am on my way home—having been warned to return if I notice any more symptoms.

The next day my ears are worse and my lips are swollen. Whether it is denial on my part I cannot say because though Eddie is at work, I still feel confident driving. Returning safely to the same medical facility, I'm somewhat taken aback by a staff member's reaction as I explain that my bottom lip is double in size compared to how it usually looks—extending down into my chin, as though I have two lower lips—one above the other. "We don't count that as swollen", I'm told with curt, dismissive, unmistakable authority. "It only counts if it swells straight out—not downward". Really? I don't think so! Excess fluid is excess fluid, regardless of where it accumulates, my non-medically-trained, but logical mind shouts in deafening silence others can't hear—but startlingly loud back at me.

After further evaluation, my steroids are increased and home I go. Disconcertingly, the lip swelling and throat constriction not only continue—but increase enough to ring that little concern bell in my head that warns it is time to return to the medical facility. Looking up at me with dismissive recognition, as though this visit is superfluous, the registrant informs me, (with all the attitude of an eye-rolling teenager who, rather than maturing, perfected the technique into adulthood), that this is my third visit in three days. Biting my tongue to refrain from retorting, "What business is it of yours?", I ignore the inappropriate comment from a receptionist and take a seat in the now all-too-familiar waiting room—hoping it won't be long before my name is called—mispronounced or not.

When the same practitioner I've had in the past walks into the exam room, he throws his arms up in the air—his frustration unconcealed. Stating he doesn't know what else he can do for me, I read more annoyance than compassion in his over-dramatic, tight-lipped, dismissive and unprofessional verbiage—particularly when he concludes the visit by offering me a sedative to "relax me". I have my analytical brain cells to silently compliment for kicking in when they do. Clearly his cavalier attitude and inability to recognize the gravity of what could be life-threatening symptoms are disconcerting—but I, for one, am not about to leave this potential reality unaddressed. "No, doctor, my intent is to get to the bottom of these PHYSICAL symptoms—with an appropriate protocol that will make them stop—NOW!"

Days later, listening to one of my established physicians detail the emergency department notes faxed to him from the facility I'd just been evaluated at, it is with disgusted disbelief that I realize the notes are not mine—but those of another patient! Informing me that I will have to discontinue the steroids I'm currently on—prior to admission for the cranial biopsy the emergency room doctor recommended for the headaches I complained of, I can feel my face tip forward as my jaw drops in astonishment. Temporarily speechless, it is in surprised silence that I listen as he continues, referencing my left-sided jaw and shoulder pain, in addition to abnormal blood work results. My ankles are reported as not swollen and my abdomen as soft—neither of which were examined. Now I've had it! With the determination of a ravenous animal teased by food, I am beyond containing myself a moment longer. "Excuse me—how can that be?", I ask what I know is a rhetorical question of this physician totally innocent of what occurred. "I never had a headache, shoulder pain or blood work drawn!" The open-mouthed, wide-eyed gape on his face reveals thoughts that corroborate mine, even before his voice can verbalize them—that the chart he received under my name really belongs to another patient. Silently I swallow my disgust, but not the unspoken question I can't shake from my mind—is there any doubt why misdiagnosis occurs, with inexcusable carelessness such as this?

Frustrating and security-robbing as that situation was, I choose to focus on more positive medical experiences. As potent and toxic as the infusions may have been, infiltrating my veins hour by hour, minute by minute, second by second, their indisputable positive effects far superseded any reluctance to continue them. If the next three-and-a-half weeks aren't justification of the quality of life change this medication provides, I don't know what is. With pain relief beyond description, I no longer cry in my sleep throughout the night whenever I move as little as an inch. Sobs that previously awakened Eddie from a deep, almost impenetrable visit with the sandman are now non-existent. No longer embarrassed by loud, involuntary moaning which I was unable to stifle from others, whenever getting in and out of cars, or up and down from church pews, I currently feel as close to "my normal" as I can remember—and I'm loving life! My miracle drug has kicked in. At this point, what's not to love?

The next morning, though an inarguably questionable winter weather driving day, we make the decision not to cancel a brunch with some of our closest friends—friends we have known for decades. As we sit comfortably around the table sharing memories and conversations only years of friendship can resurrect, I can't help but notice difficulty in enunciating my words. Not only do I recognize hoarseness, but about three hours into the visit I feel a tightness—like an elastic band with tension on it is constricting the back of my throat! Coincidentally, the weather continues to worsen making it easier for all of us to call it a day—which, based on these latest unshared physical developments, I have no hesitation doing.

Really scared, my only consolation as we get into the car is that our paramedic friend, Keith, is driving. Trying to make my voice as nonchalant as possible, I ask him a question that is out-of-character for me. "I've always been curious", my deceptive intentions materialize into transparent words, "when you transport patients by ambulance, and a breathing tube is inserted, do you anesthetize?" my now even-hoarser voice croaks.

With three alarming pairs of eyes shot in my direction, the suspicious questions and comments are almost too much to keep up with. "Are you all right"? "Do you want to go straight to the hospital?", "Should we call 911?", etc. It is like Denise is looking through a window into my brain when she combines the question I asked with my unspoken fears as she asserts, "Eileen NEVER asks a question as medically specific as that—unless there is a good reason"—and she is right. So much for trying to come across as casual—I should have known better, given how well they know me.

Because I want to talk to my doctor first, I spend the rest of the ride trying to convince them that I'm fine. No one is buying it, however. Concerned eyes reflect back at me from the rearview mirror, while the others attempt to engage me in continual and, what I know to be purposeful conversation.

As soon as we get home, I quickly provide Eddie with more details regarding what is going on. By now, my breathing has become labored—clearly, I'm in trouble. At the same time, as far as I'm concerned, three strikes and you're out! I REFUSE to return to the same medical facility.

Though somewhat embarrassed to go elsewhere, after being treated by previous staff as though some of my visits were superfluous, my gut feeling is that I am in a life-threatening situation—and I'm scared! Without his awareness, I look across the room at the husband I love more than life itself and realize that between him, my children and grandchildren, there is no choice—I need competent medical help and I need it now!

Selecting a very reputable facility, I hesitantly share with the triage nurse that, based on previous recent emergency department visits for the same symptoms, I'm not sure if I should be here. Describing my current health status, I am almost taken aback by the unexpected and undisguised, worried intensity of eyes that look directly into mine—as she points to the packed-beyond-recommended-capacity waiting room, compassionately telling me that I need to be here more than anyone out there. "I have the head nurse preparing a room for you as we speak", she states with an immediacy in her voice that is impossible to conceal.

The dry, salty taste in my mouth, combined with arm hairs that stand up straight like little soldiers at attention, are my body's way of realizing—for the first time since the onset of this reaction—that I am not the only one fearing for my life. I suppose the scariest part to me, as my teeth begin to chatter noisily and uncontrollably, (much to my embarrassment), is the worry reflected back at my pooling but unspilled eyes, from experienced ones that have seen situations like mine—gone wrong.

Self-consciously trembling but unable to stop, I obediently

follow the physician's assistant through the buzzer-entry, opened door, almost too scared to think what is in store for me on the other side— but more frightened not to address such serious, potentially life-threatening symptoms.

A lab technician in cheerful, patterned cartooned scrubs enters my now-assigned, curtained off area and introduces herself to us. After verifying my identity by cross-checking my answers to her questions with information on my wristband, she ties a tourniquet on my arm and draws a few tubes of blood.

Just as she finishes shaking them, the physician's assistant returns to further question me regarding my symptoms. He then summons the physician he reports to. Collectively, they decide to call in an ear, nose and throat specialist for a consult.

When he arrives, he scopes my throat to determine if anything appears to be out of the ordinary. Though we are told everything looks fine, a few minutes later he second guesses himself, remarking that something way back at the bottom of my tongue could have represented some swelling. Unfortunately, he did not document that detail, having mentioned it subsequent to completing his section of my report.

Shortly after he exits, the physician's assistant returns with a high-dose, concentrated shot of steroids. After it is administered, I am closely monitored for several hours. Satisfied that my symptoms are responding positively, the team collectively agrees that I do not have to be admitted, (which until they share that with me, I honestly didn't even realize was under consideration). With a prescription for a hefty, pill-form steroid dose in hand, I am sent home—but not before being emphatically warned to return, should things worsen.

Within the next few days, things do worsen—but not in the way the warning was intended. Instead, from a vanity point of view, given the high steroids currently in my system—and the abnormal disfiguration they generate. Disgusted with the dramatic change, it resurrects a childhood memory I'd hoped to forget. Even at the supposedly innocent age of eight, I'm vain enough to move quickly away from the House of Mirrors reflection that transforms my already pudgy body into fatter and squattier. Opting to remain in front of the image that stretches me to several feet taller and multiple flattering inches slimmer, I want to stay here forever. But my older cousins' impatience to get to the roller coaster works to my disadvantage—awakening me from my momentary reverie as I reluctantly vacate the attraction. Clinging to the magical thinking of the little girl I still am, however, allows me to wishfully glance at my reflection in a mirror at a concession booth on the way to the next ride—only to face the disappointing reality that the image I liked best was left behind in the distortion of the House of Mirrors. For me, nothing had changed.

Fast forward to five-plus decades later, as an adult I experience a familiar disorientation—only this time one that I can't explain. Like in the House of Mirrors, my visual perception is distorted, I'm off balance and nothing is where it should be. Unlike my childhood experience, I didn't bring this on voluntarily by going to an amusement park, nor can I make it go away by exiting an attraction. Whereas everyone who entered the House of Mirrors saw the same distortion, today I am navigating in my own personal world of confusion which, no one else can see as I do—and it's a scary, insecure feeling, to say the least.

Coincidentally, I'm scheduled for an appointment with my internist next week. Looking forward to the well-timed, previously scheduled slot, I'm optimistic that this doctor I've come to trust— impeccably—will have some thoughts regarding what is going on and, more importantly, how to rectify it.

Immersed in so many other distracting responsibilities, I have little time to focus on waiting for my appointment. As a result, it seems to arrive deceptively quicker than I expected. Before I know it, I'm pumping up the volume to the oldies folk CD Eddie bought me for Christmas, loudly singing along while driving to my doctor's—confident that my tone-deafness offends no one, given I'm the only one within earshot—and I'm not musically gifted enough to recognize it anyway.

Continuing to sing in a voice others have asked me—in not so many words—"why bother?", I'm again feeling nostalgic as my solo sing-a-long resurrects another memory I haven't rekindled in decades. At the innocent age of ten, I had no clue what "tone-deaf" meant. Instead, I sung my heart out during car rides with my dad, brother Al, Auntie Helen and Uncle Al—feeling very comfortable and not in the least bit self-conscious doing so. No one ever told me I sounded awful, so why would I even begin to think that? Given the complimentary words my loving and positive aunt used every time I chose a particularly touching song—words that still remain in my heart decades later—(and never fail to make my lips curve into a warm, reminiscent smile whenever my mind provides me the opportunity to re-visit that coveted chamber—the one that houses memories both of her and the valuable lessons she instilled in me)— there was no reason to believe otherwise. Certainly, I didn't see anyone covering their ears. Then again, maybe they should have. That way I wouldn't have had the confidence to try out for the children's Christmas Eve Church Choir—but fortunately, (or unfortunately, depending on whose ears were subjected to this decision), I did! I wanted to be in it so badly—as did all of my closest friends.

I know people who insist that things always seem bigger,

better, etc. when viewed through childhood memories—but inarguably, (at least in my mind), there are times they really were. I can still visualize the old, ornately-decorated, breathtakingly-beautiful church—just the thought of which resurrects the unforgettably pleasa0nt scent, (stored in memory banks I would have thought were non-existent by now—yet incredibly still retrievable, more than half a century later), of aged wood from which it was constructed. In contrast to the activity level of the weekend services our family regularly attended, the day my mind transports me back to is unusually quiet—empty except for our small audition group climbing the steep steps to the choir loft. That, in itself, is exciting. It is the first time most of us have ever been on a spiral stair case, as the loft is typically reserved exclusively for the adult choir. Feeling awkward, initially, as I've never seen stairs that are wide on one side and very narrow on the other, I'm not quite sure how to negotiate them, so I decide to take the safe route—stepping on the wide sections while clinging to the thick wooden rail as I tenuously climb higher and higher. With every creak, our unsureness morphs into anticipation. Reaching the top, we look over the massive rail at an impressive perspective of the church that, to-date, was nonexistent—at least to us. With the sun shining through the breathtakingly beautiful stained-glassed windows, we can't help but notice the pews look further away than usual—as do the statues. Actually, it is next to impossible to make out their porcelain faces at such a distance.

At one point, I ask myself how choir members can even hear the priest during Mass from our distant, bird's eye perch—a question "myself" has no opportunity to answer, with that thought put on hold due to the arrival of Sister-I'm-Sorry-I've-Long-Since-Forgotten- Your-Name. But trust me—HER we can hear! As she quickly heads to the piano situated at the front of the loft, she instructs us to select one of the cushy, red velvet chairs assembled in rows. Telling us she is going to choose some familiar Christmas songs to sing, just to get a feel for where we are at, (whatever that means), so far other than doing so before

Halloween, which seems date-inappropriate to me, the audition really doesn't sound too challenging. And as far as singing Christmas songs prematurely, I suppose it is necessary to allow enough practice time before the big night.

Unaware of my musical "disability", I confidently sing "Away in a Manger" with enthusiastic volume. Oops! Big mistake! When the nun says, "SOMEONE is off", I look around the dimly lit loft at all present thinking hmm, I wonder who it could be—which soon changes to a fear that I, personally, will find out.

Row by row, as we sing, she squeezes in front of each of us with her hand cupped behind her ear and bent in our direction, in an effort to locate the off-key voice. My insecurity escalates big-time when she reaches my row—the last row—without having identified the "offender". Uh-oh, there are only three of us left—What if it is ME?

(Disconcertingly, even decades later as I share this experience, it makes me cringe to still recall, so vividly, the ripples of self-doubt that suddenly replaced previously-naïve confidence—in a little girl unexpectedly faced with the real world—and the challenges it can undeservedly present.) But back to the audition: Oh, how I want to be a part of The Children's Midnight Mass Christmas Eve Choir with all my friends. I want to wear the long red and white robe with the wide sleeves and hold a candle while parishioners look up from their pews to see where the beautiful singing is coming from— and I'm bound and determined to do so. But how? Sister has listened to everyone but me and no one was singled out as off-key. I have to do something creative—and fast! As a last-ditch effort to be with my friends on a night I know I will never forget, when she gets to me I mouth the words instead of singing. Hoping that whispers can't be off-key I give it a try and, believe it or not, it works! Returning to the piano, she only mumbles once under her breath when we resume singing, (which I do with all my heart),— insisting that someone is still off-key.

Though none of us is accustomed to being up at midnight, we are all too excited to feel tired when the long-awaited Christmas Eve choir performance finally arrives, (analogous to how adrenalin magically kicking in at a friend's sleep-over, when guests stay up all night). Excitement intensifies with every step as our feet pitter-patter up the creaky old stairs—just a little faster than they are supposed to—making clicking sounds in our shiny black patent leather dress shoes. In contrast to the otherwise dark choir loft, our holiday-scrubbed, deceptively-cherubic faces are aglow from the candles we hold in front of them. Parishioners in the beautifully- decorated church—exuding the intoxicatingly festive scents of Christmas—smile appreciatively up at us from their shoulder-to- shoulder packed pews as we sing our little hearts out. And you know what? No one seems to notice—or care—that "someone" is off- key. It was obviously a night that, to this day, I've never forgotten!

Now back to my current reality—Frustrated beyond words with my inability to find a physician able to resolve these serious and scary allergic reactions, I initiate an online search. Identifying one who treats adults—a challenge in itself, considering the majority I come across specialize in pediatrics—I contact his office. When I do, the doctor humbly informs me that though he would be very willing to see me, he knows of a physician far more experienced with the specific allergies I describe—and I welcome his honest advice.

Before meeting the specialist, I am asked to detail 0 my history to two residents who take copious notes, momentarily reverting me back to my own college days when I filled large notebooks—quoting professors as close to verbatim as possible within those skinny, college-ruled lines—fearful if I missed one word it would be the answer to an exam question. During the history taking, I mention that I had an anaphylactic reaction to an infusion and have been adversely reacting ever since. When I do, one looks at me with the innocence of wide-eyed child accused of something they did not do. "What does anaphylaxis mean?", she asks. Resisting the urge to overreact by pointing out that this is one of the most critical conditions someone in the medical field should be readily able to identify, (even while still a student), I opt to use this moment as a teaching opportunity. After all, it really isn't her fault—she slipped through the cracks. However, in my opinion, lives can't be at risk because of avoidable slippages such as this. To get to the level she is at without mastering understanding of such a crucial concept is inexcusable—not to mention dangerous! Though only able to answer her question through firsthand experience, rather than medical textbook explanations—it's a start—but not sufficient. Before leaving, I confidentially mention to a staff member that I noticed uncertainty regarding anaphylaxis when interviewed by one of the students. I was thanked profusely for bringing it to her attention and told such feedback is invaluable in determining curriculum deficits. My hope in mentioning it is that another patient won't experience the danger and fear of having to save their own life—because an anaphylactic reaction was missed. (As far as I'm concerned, everyone should know the signs of such a dangerous reaction. It could save a life!)

Now back to the students' findings following their history taking: After verbally regurgitating their notes to the doctor they train under as I wait for them to reappear in the exam room, they return with a white-coat-clad, immediately-likable physician whom I meet for the first time.

After reading the residents' notes she asks a few additional questions, examines my lips, (which are slightly swollen) and, with that, concludes her physical assessment. When I try to show her my gums, where the swelling is even more prevalent, she disregards my attempt—telling me she doesn't need to see them—indicating that she has a handle on what I am experiencing. She then adds another antihistamine to what I'm currently taking and schedules a subsequent appointment in two weeks.

Before leaving the exam room, she asks the students to get a picture of my swollen lips and, after assuring me that this new prescription will rectify the situation, we are on our way.

Disconcertingly, despite the added medications my symptoms don't improve in the least. Once again, I'm insecure about having to make decisions I'm not trained to do—i.e. saving my own life by deciding if I should up my steroids, go to the Emergency Department, etc.

With the stress of these responsibilities I am not medically trained to confidently monitor, the two-week wait seems like an eternity. Meanwhile the burning itch has reached a state of intolerable beyond words. I have all I can do to prevent myself from scratching my skin off from its intensity, which in addition to itching, hurts. My body is riddled with marks it never wore before. Their irregularly-shaped blobs are numerous enough to create a connect-the-dots picture on a canvas I never asked to wear—but involuntarily do. With no other recourse, I continue to swallow antihistamines like candy—but without the palette-pleasing pleasure candy affords. My life revolves around this to-date uncontrolled disease, rather than the disease revolving around how I treat it. My world—as I knew it—has changed, significantly—and I ache for the old one back. There are no words to describe the Hell I currently reside in—nor is there a way to even begin to explain it to others.

When the appointment date finally arrives, I can almost feel my invisible-to-me heart sigh with a smile of relief when my now-familiar immunologist enters the exam room. Her face defined by a welcoming smile, she queries how I am doing and seems surprised to learn the symptoms persist. Finding her confused by some of my questions, I note that she scrolls back and forth on my computerized chart, re-familiarizing her memory with details of our last visit, which makes sense given the large patient load she must have—in a specialized field with so few doctors.

Mentioning that my lips continue to swell intermittently, she responds that they aren't at the moment. Yes, my non-verbal dialect shares only with myself—as I said, "intermittently".

She then instructs me to take pictures of the swelling before returning to her, once again in two weeks. According to her, she needs to see the swelling, herself, which she claims she has not. Perhaps she has forgotten that she asked her students to take pictures of the atypical size she noted at my first visit—which they neglected to do.

When I ask her if a documented note from my primary care physician who has seen them will suffice, I'm told that isn't enough. Frustrated that she never got photos of the ones she asked her students to take—and that she doesn't have that request documented—I begin to question, in my own mind, whether she possesses the level of competency my case requires. However, giving her the benefit of the doubt, I stop at the reception desk on my way out and schedule the appointment she instructs me to make—a decision I later regret.

You know that stunned-silent feeling one experiences when someone says exactly the opposite thing you were expecting to hear? That speechless state of confusion overwhelms me at my next visit as I listen in disbelief to the immunologist tell me I needn't come back. Am I hearing things, my mind asks itself in silence?

Momentarily taken off guard, once I regain my composure the logical side of me asks whether I really want to continue seeing a physician who doesn't recognize the need for me to return. In a confused patient-fog I inform the receptionist, on my way out, that scheduling another appointment is unnecessary.

Like a hopelessly trapped zoo visitor who accidentally fell into a ferocious animal's cage, I'm petrified and unsure where to turn next. While inarguably the fate of the unfortunate want-to-be-spectator is more immediate and potentially fatal, contending with uncontrolled anaphylactic symptoms, on a daily basis, can result in the same demise.

Lost in further thought, my mind questions how one tiny white pill—or in my case, several—can help so much yet distort my body into someone almost unrecognizable? It disturbs me beyond words to admit—even to myself—that, at the moment—these little white pills that have literally robbed me of my femininity are also my lifeline. Controlling, or at least lessening the itching, lip swelling, chest tightness and throat constriction, they are a necessity I can't afford to do without.

Though magically, (or not so), causing the pain due to swelling in various areas of my body to partially subside, I ask myself why the treatment couldn't also take the swelling away, deflating my grossly distorted body like a child's balloon from a party they had attended far-too-many-days-ago to retain its air. Unlike the child, at times dissolved in disappointed tears, it would be a blessing if my swollen areas deflated—as though popped by a pin—never to inflate again. Disconcertingly, at the moment no one seems to have figured out how to make this happen. At best, the little white pills remain my life-saving "candy", despite their unflattering side-effects. Though every immunologist I've seen—to date—assures me I won't have to live with these symptoms the rest of my life, nothing they have done to address this nightmare has proven their words to be true.

In desperation, I once again resort to the internet—searching, without any recommendations, (as I'd exhausted the few in this specialty that my other physicians knew of), for another immunologist. Impressed with the credentials of one in particular, I immediately jot down the office number provided. Though she is located four hours away, the drive would be more than worth it if it meant finding a solution to these horrific, continual and scary reactions. Besides, ideally this specialist will provide an effective protocol and share it with a local immunologist in my home state— from where future treatments can be dispensed. Regardless, one thing is certain—if I want to live, I've got to do something!

Feeling a little like a focused teeny bopper unable to put down her phone, I punch in the telephone number of the physician's office. The difference is calls generated by teens are often related to something carefree and fun—trust me, there is no enjoyment in trying to beat the clock in order to save one's life!

Not surprisingly, specialized as she has been described, this doctor is so busy her staff is booking appointments a month in advance—an eternity from where I stand. Desperate, I detail some of my symptoms to the receptionist who, though she books my appointment in thirty days, promises to place me on a cancellation list, should a slot become available sooner.

Before our conversation ends, I'm told the nurse would like to speak to me. Encountering a friendly, but unmistakably concerned voice on the other end—evidenced by the number of details she requests—she assures me that the physician I will be seeing has successfully treated other cases like mine and will definitely be able to help. Before our conversation ends, I tell her I look forward to meeting her—a sentiment she shares back to me. Silently I ask myself what distractions I can possibly come up with to get through the next thirty days of potentially life-threatening symptoms—until my appointment with this specialist whom, though I've never met, I already have more confidence in than she has had an opportunity to prove I should. But I need to cling to something and, at the moment, she is the best show in town. More accurately, the only one.

Shocked to see the name and number of her office light my phone, just two days later, I answer expecting to be instructed to forward medical records. Much to my unexpected relief, I'm asked if I am available to come in tomorrow. Am I available? I'll jump through hoops to be there, I think to myself.

With Eddie and I in deep, thought-provoking, serious conversation, the long ride passes much quicker than I would have expected. Like my first visits with the other new immunologists, optimism sends rivers through the tributaries of blood flowing throughout my body, praying this will be the one—the one with a solution to this anaphylactic nightmare.

Checking in at the front desk, I thank the staff for getting me in so quickly, despite the cancellation list which I am sure offered much competition from others vying for those coveted and rare slots that open unexpectedly. I'm told that their cancellation list is prioritized by patient severity, which explains the expediency demonstrated in fitting me in. Recalling the nurse's detailed phone interview, I have no doubt she actually triages through her questioning—determining which patients need to be seen first. Before I have the opportunity to analyze their impressive scheduling "wait list" system any further, her nurse calls my name and ushers us into a little room where vitals are taken and an even more comprehensive interview ensues. Concluding by saying the doctor is "chomping at the bit" to meet me, after reading the notes, she leads us to her office.

Reminiscent of an old library, the kind our dad used to take us to, the scent of the leather volumes lining three of her walls is intoxicating—in a good way. The last time I remember this pleasant aroma, I was about five, clinging to my dad's hand—welcoming the security it offered as we walked between library book shelves on glass floors. As a child, I was afraid the glass could break and we would fall through, whereas my adult logic knows better, remembering how thick the frosted, translucent glass floors really were.

The fourth wall of the physician's office is virtually wallpapered with medical degrees—not only a tribute to her ability but a visual that makes me secure.

Nicely attired in a crisply ironed shirt and matching printed skirt, layered with an open white coat with her name embroidered on it, she exudes a casual but unmistakable professionalism that I immediately find relaxing. Seated at a massive cherry desk in the middle of the room, she stands and introduces herself as soon as we are within shaking-hands-distance.

Following some small talk regarding our long ride and what route we took, she loses no time getting right down to business, focusing primarily on the excessive number of autoimmune diseases I have, and have had, over a period of so many years. Reaching for one of her leather-bound volumes, that she stores at her fingertips, it would be impossible to overlook the frequent use it gets, judging by its wrinkled, yellowed pages—with bookmarks Interspersed throughout.

Flipping through it as I simultaneously respond to her more detailed questions regarding the autoimmune diseases, she nods her head up and down the entire time, indicating familiarity with what I'm describing—not only verbally but through her body language as well. Clearly, she has heard this before and, more importantly, knows how to treat it. For the first time since challenged by aggressive daily anaphylaxis, Eddie and I are encouraged.

According to her, what I have is something with a simple solution. When put in those terms, after the severity of what I've experienced over the past several months, red flags erupt from my skeptical brain cells—while my optimistic ones shove them out of the way like an older sibling overpowering a younger one. At least give her a chance, the logical part of my thinking silently shouts, relieved to hear it more loudly than the doubtful side.

As the silent but distracting logical and emotional thinking battle subsides, it is easier to concentrate on what the physician is saying as she confidently prescribes shots to counteract the reaction, via a medication virtually no one reacts to. She continues by explaining that this drug, administered in an outpatient hospital setting, has been highly effective in eliminating the same symptoms I'm experiencing—and she wants me to start immediately.

Optimistically, we arrive at the hospital two days later at eleven A.M., for the first of a series that will continue for seven to eight months. Following each injection, I will be monitored for a few hours to assure no adverse reactions occur.

Sitting in the small but adequate waiting room listening to the bubbling sound of the corner water cooler situated next to a tower of cone-shaped, unused paper cups—the kind Italian ice often comes in—I can hear another patient being instructed as to the process that occurs when given the same medication I came here for. With ears listening as though they are on steroids, my curiosity peaks with every word I intentionally overhear, especially when the patient queries her regarding adverse reactions. Much like my doctor's response, her answer is reassuring—not only to the understandably curious patient she is currently addressing, but to me as well. "Only a miniscule number of people would ever react to this virtually benign medication", she asserts with confidence that puts me at ease. "But what if I did?" he further probes. "Then we'd just have to keep you", she matter-of-factly replies—once again with the implication that there is no need to worry as this was not going to happen. Did I really have to overhear THAT question and more importantly—answer, I ask myself as my worry wart brain cells go into overdrive?

Before further violation of HIPAA (Health Insurance Portability and Accountability Act of 1996) occurs, providing me with additional intimate specifics of this gentleman's case, another nurse leads me to a comfortable-looking vinyl recliner where my own treatment will be administered.

Once I am situated in the chair, a warm blanket is unfolded and placed over me, covering my body from shoulders to my toes. Feeling so good in contrast to the slightly chilly room, it entices me to appreciatively snuggle up in it—like a child being tucked in by her mom. A far less cushy, but still very doable side chair is provided for Eddie so that he can sit next to me while we both challenge the computer to Scrabble—an enjoyable distraction we frequently rely on to make time pass during long medical procedures.

Within a few minutes, my nurse is disinfecting my arms with alcohol wipes, then injecting a shot of the prescribed medication into each one.

Even the challenge presented trying to make a word out of our all-vowel rack of letters is not perplexing enough to camouflage the chest constriction that manifests within ten minutes of injection. Trying to play the mind-over-matter card doesn't work, either. Tears I refuse to let fall lubricate the inside of my eyes, generated by disappointment—crushed that the "solution" I had such high hopes for,—isn't.

Staunch, stubborn and ego-challenged on my second office visit, my physician's "attempt" at communication is tight-lipped and over-confident. Her dismissive body language is inarguably anger-driven, annoyed with ME because her recommended treatment didn't work—and, in fact, triggered an adverse reaction. Part of me is convinced she is angrier at herself—but projecting it in a more socially acceptable, ego-stroking way—onto me!

What was once described as an "easy solution" couldn't be farther from the truth. Unable to accept my body's inability to safely tolerate her recommended protocol, she arrogantly insists that I repeat the regiment that caused the adverse reaction in the first place.

Sarcastically, when I explain the chest tightness I experienced within ten minutes of being injected, she flippantly throws an arm up into the air, telling me that isn't considered a reaction because it isn't something I could show her—nor prove. Excuse me? Am I supposed to try to get a picture of that, too? Really? And, if so, how?

Continuing on in a holier-than-thou, condescending tone, she adamantly asserts that the drug she prescribed couldn't cause chest constriction. Adding insult to injury, she demonstrates an even more demeaning, unprofessional attitude when she says, "You know what? I'm going to put "anxiety" down as your diagnosis." Like I'm surprised! Her treatment was not only unsuccessful and potentially harmful—but her ego too inflated to accept that. Is there any question why misdiagnosis statistics remain unacceptably high with such close-minded thinking on the part of SOME practitioners? Fortunately, they are not the norm, but disconcertingly, they still influence the numbers—and, more importantly, patients' lives.

Unconvinced—but with no documentation at my fingertips to otherwise prove that chest constriction could be a side effect subsequent to injection of the medication I received, I make a mental note to research that possibility, in detail, when I get home. (Ironically, but supporting my supposition, when I do it lists chest constriction as one of the first possible adverse reactions to this drug.)

It embarrasses me to admit that under duress, before leaving I make the obligatory appointment for a return visit that she instructs me to do. Even more incredulous, I schedule the asap second round of shots—the same injections that initiated the reaction. While I may feel I'm given no choice at the time—and I do—there is no excuse for allowing intimidation to control such a serious decision. What if I react again? It doesn't require a medical degree to educate one's self that subsequent reactions are often more serious—and sometimes fatal!

Do I hear a familiar ring here? Suddenly red flags unfurl in the still-rebounding, demeaned cells of my brain as it occurs to me that Dr. Rosenbaum and the close-minded physician who insisted that I continue a drug I was adversely reacting to were trained during the same medical school era—the only difference is that the author recognizes it and has adjusted his way of practicing medicine to avoid the damage such thinking can result in. With fire igniting through my veins, too continuous for any hoses to extinguish, this image on my mind's T.V. screen is the only "anxiety-driven" aspect of my medical mystery!

I feel like a jerk! How stupid can I be to sit back and allow multiple immunologists I've seen dismiss potentially life-threatening symptoms that they are unable to diagnose and/or cure? Why didn't I demand more from them—like subsequent referrals to those who potentially could?

Instead, I wasn't demonstrative enough when given inaccurate and unacceptable theories such as: "Sometimes a patient's throat can FEEL tight—like it's closing—when it really isn't", (ooh, too serious a symptom to take a chance on, don't you think? What if the PATIENT is right and the doctor isn't in this case?). What about not pursuing why Emergency Department reports of another patient were transferred to a different facility under MY name— most particularly the one that stated I should immediately wean down on my steroids in preparation for brain surgery, (which I was never informed of nor, thankfully, required)—due to the headaches I presented with? Considering I never had nor complained of a headache during my entire work-up, I find such inaccuracy on the part of the medical staff totally unacceptable—particularly with the potentially unnecessary and serious surgery recommended due to careless combining of two patients' charts. Disconcerting as this is I have no control over the fact that it occurred, but I can take responsibility for my own actions—and, in truth, I disappointed myself. To allow this without following up with a letter and/or call to the facility where the misinformation was generated was my mistake. Though it would not change things for me, it could have a major impact on future patients—especially if pointing out the error resulted in a more effective system to prevent accidentally switching patients' charts. In retrospect, it was also irresponsible of me not to question those notes that stated in writing that I looked fine, reading a book on a gurney, when I had no book; or why blood work results were included in my chart when no blood was drawn. Didn't it even occur to me to ask how the physician I saw knew my abdomen was "soft" when he never touched it? Does it get any scarier than this? Not to use it as a cop out—but I will—patients are often far too ill, (myself included), to make anything besides getting better their priority. Trust me, the last thing on their minds is using already depleted energy to call institutions or start letter writing campaigns addressing non-effectivity in medical treatment, which, in some cases involuntarily enables misdiagnosis.

Though I'm not certain where to go from here, one thing I AM certain of—after alone time for contemplation with Eddie—is it will NOT be back to the physician I just left. She's history! When she gets back to her office tomorrow, my voicemail will be on her machine, cancelling both my intimidation-generated future office visit and up-and-coming infusion appointment. Contrary as I realize this decision is to her advice, it is my body—and my choice. Actually, as I see it, there IS no choice.

Picking my own far-too-picked brain, I once again resort to depending on the computer to search for a new immunologist—and, as in the past, my choices are limited. Not only is the field so specialized, but the ages of patients they treat—which, in most cases, means I'm too old. However, I do find one that treats all ages and is conveniently located in my state. Calling her office, I explain my predicament to her medical associate. After running it by her, she agrees to give it a shot. Not having met her, I'm already impressed by the lack of doctor–god attitude she demonstrates. While her response makes no promises that she will solve this mystery, eluding to a truth I wish all practitioners were open-minded enough to admit to their patients, that they aren't infallible, at the same time she conveys the feeling that she will do her very best—which offers hope to a patient who really could use some at this point. It is with refreshing optimism that I schedule my first appointment.

Sitting in her office a few weeks later, I detail my symptoms and answer any questions she has regarding them. I am honest about how many physicians I've consulted and facilities I've been to. My respect for her grows by the minute when, with humility, she admits that my case is beyond the limits of most immunologists—but that she does know a hospital that specializes in reactions as serious as the one I am experiencing.

Though distance is involved, at this point I will try ANYTHING. Not only is my quality of life incredibly compromised, but more importantly, I feel at risk—despite carrying an epi pen and antihistamines wherever I go. While to date I've been able to monitor and address the continuing daily anaphylactic symptoms with the tools at my disposal, what if I have an episode during which they don't work? Certainly, I was prepared during our last blizzard by stocking up on steroids because the storm was predicted to be severe—actually one which would prevent travel— but suppose I didn't consider that ahead of time and ran out. These are not decisions I should be responsible for—but if I'm not, who will be? As much as I know I shouldn't allow myself to give in and fall asleep in the middle of the night if I'm reacting with anaphylaxis, what if the sandman wins over chest tightening and/or itching? Despite antihistamines, epi pens and 911, what if they prove ineffective? I've awaken to scary throat constriction before—does that mean it will happen again—and, if so, will it be in time to administer something to counteract it? Isn't it enough to experience these life-threatening daily symptoms—without having to control their management? Yet, as these concerns clog my head relentlessly, I can't ignore them—nor should I.

Appreciative as I am for the recommendation to a facility she has so much confidence in, I must admit a twinge of regret that the doctor suggesting it is unable to take over my case. I can't think of many I would rather have managing it. Though logically I'm convinced my life depends on seeing the practitioner most experienced in treating a persistent and atypical allergic reaction such as mine, just knowing that this physician—perceptive and humble enough to recognize the need to refer me elsewhere intends to remain involved—is encouraging.

A combination of optimism and trepidation are in contention, challenging each other in their efforts to overtake my thoughts as we check into our hotel the night before my early-morning appointment at the facility our local immunologist recommended—and, unfortunately, trepidation appears to be winning. Trying to will the negative away, I do my best to focus on what I was told when being referred here, especially the part about how many other patients—who were unsuccessfully treated for unrelenting anaphylaxis at various institutions—found resolution from the care and experience provided at this hospital. With that thought, after a long and arduous day, I take a lengthy and relaxing bath and sink into the comfort of the hotel's invitingly soft, pillow-top mattress as I wrap myself into a snuggly down comforter cocoon. Considering the depth of my sleep, when the hotel's wake-up call rings close to my ear I feel startled—as though from a far-away planet. However, no longer apprehensive, I'm optimistically excited at the prospect of what I have to gain today—an answer to the perplexing nightmare I've been involuntarily living.

Following a quick breakfast, we head for the facility where my appointment is scheduled. Handing in the pre-completed form that was mailed to me, I'm escorted to a doctor's office—but much to my disappointment, not the one I was told I would be seeing today. Informing me that she will be conducting allergy testing to determine the things I am sensitive to, she further assures me that she works directly with the doctor I was originally scheduled to see. Continuing on, she queries me regarding any gaps in the written history I provided. True to her word, she administers a few shots and sends me out to the waiting room where she periodically checks my arm for possible reactions. Within minutes I exhibit large, raised, blistering mosquito-bite-like itchy bumps—and even bigger hives. Because of this, an appointment with the physician I was originally referred to is made. Consequently, I will be returning within the month.

Waiting for the scheduled slot went quickly, probably due to the many other doctors' appointments that distracted me during the interim. Sitting in the office of this renown immunologist who has every reason to have attitude—but refreshingly doesn't—her down-to-earth demeanor is so impressive one is comfortably at ease from the moment she meets her. After describing my symptoms, she prescribes an antihistamine far stronger those I've used to-date, which I'm instructed to add to my already copious regiment. I also learn that the shots I received were administered much too aggressively—and that they should have been introduced far more gradually, increasing them a little each time until the goal dosage was attained—which is the approach she intends to take.

Before leaving, infusion dates are scheduled for the preferred, lower dosage amount she recommends initiating administration at. With each dose, I will be under constant one-on-one nursing supervision for the entire day—with an allergy-trained physician available throughout my visit. Unfortunately, upon my return—gradual as the drips are—I still experience adverse and increasing reactions with each one, to the point of scary. Observing the impossible-to-miss crash carts strategically positioned at my bedside, I pray they won't be necessary.

I'm especially unnerved when one doctor has to stop the infusion each time my chest tightens, my throat constricts and the itchiness begins—only to re-start it when it resolves. Despite his encouragement that I can do this, I know my body and I have my doubts. What if the symptoms get too severe to stop? I don't even want to go there!

Meanwhile, life at home, between infusions, goes on. With double and triple chins reflecting back at me in ugly rolls from the bathroom mirror, it once again disgusts me to think that the high dose steroids which I still take are responsible for nothing more than disfiguring me, (a slight frustration-generated exaggeration as they also help with the pain). Momentarily, my mind allows me to contrast these negative rolls to the positive ones I remember from when I was a little girl—those that were not attached to my body. Even many decades later I'm still impressed by the stairs of grass my memory doesn't allow me to forget—and I hope it never will. Situated at the front of a local school yard my dad used to take us to, unlike the rolls I now see I loved those. Rolling down them was a positive experience—one I'd give anything to resurrect with my dad. It was such fun to stretch out as far as I could, arms peaked way above my head—hands clasped into a point as I rolled down nature's staircase.

Trust me, the exuberant child I describe from the past, who clung to her dad's hand making him run to keep up with her as we approached the school yard, has transformed into an adult disappointed with the ineffectiveness of this grossly disfiguring medication—as far as curing the anaphylaxis that results in rolls far less pleasurable than those she remembers from childhood. Inarguably, going off of it is not an option because though it doesn't cure the anaphylaxis, in truth it controls it enough to prevent me from dying—so referring to it as ineffective is unfair and impatient on my part.

Disappointingly, the grass stairs no longer exist, (undoubtedly to the groundskeepers' relief as I can't imagine mowing them)—which is probably why I've never seen any like them since. But thankfully, my mind allows me to re-visit them in the privacy of my thoughts. As it does, this and other priceless memories cause my eyes to fill, bittersweetly—

grateful to have them but saddened that they have become just that—memories—rather than in-person experiences still occurring.

CHAPTER TWELVE

A Physician Who Has Earned My Respect Forever!

"It's not so much the journey that's important; as is the way that we treat those we encounter and those around us, along the way."

—Jeremy Aldana

Salivating from the intoxicating aromas of breakfast cooking— the sizzling bacon that my mind can almost visualize shrinking as the grill spits its hot grease in all directions, the toast that pops up high in the air when it turns a perfect golden brown but not burnt, the coffee whose irresistible scent infiltrates my nostrils—enticingly reminding me I haven't had my first cup of the day, yet—fresh baked muffins with its crevices drinking up the butter it is smeared with, etc., the familiarity of this local coffee shop is such that the waitresses have the orders of regular customers committed to memory.

Frequenting it with my daily church group friends, the comradery is comforting and, today of all days, I don't want to leave. Apprehension infiltrates my veins from head-to-toe at the thought of why I have to vacate the restaurant early—to travel out of state to an immunology appointment I'm not feeling optimistic about. After multiple attempts at desensitization to the medication I originally adversely reacted to more than a year ago—with life- threatening symptoms—there has been no improvement. Instead, with every infusion in an attempt to allow my body to acclimate to it, I'm worse—worse to the point that I'm afraid to have another, petrified that the crash cart equipment strategically positioned directly by my side, during these procedures, will be used—on me!

Fortunately, today involves no desensitization. Actually, I have an appointment scheduled with my physician. It isn't even in the same town or location, but at the medical facility where I was originally privileged enough to meet this incredibly competent physician

Today is the second day of a forecasted oppressive heat wave and trust me, the weatherman didn't get it wrong! Barely able to breathe the 94-degree hot, humid air that fogs my glasses in the short twelve-foot walk from our cab to the building, the cool air conditioning is a relief words can't describe once the motion-detected, automatic door to the medical center opens, with its welcoming frigid blast enticing us to enter.

Watching the numbered floors light up, my mind wanders involuntarily as I impatiently look for the eighth floor to illuminate, a signal that the elevator has reached our destination.

While multiple physicians have done their best to alleviate the dangerous and, at times, life-threatening allergic symptoms I've experienced daily—for more than a year and a half—I am still disconcertingly aware that I have been—and remain—

responsible in many ways for saving my own life. With no permanent solution to-date for the continuous reactions, like my doctors, I, too, need to know when to administer symptomatic and crucial treatment. After all, they come on at any time, day and/or night—and certainly I can't expect physicians to be by my side, for more than a year, 24/7 monitoring them. Though vigilant, as in the past I still remain insecure determining which medicines—and when—I should be using based on the presenting problem. In addition, I have dosage amounts to decide on my own, after considering the severity—ever conscious of the importance of remaining "on top of my game" and ahead of the symptoms.

Fortunately, the life-saving array of antihistamines my physicians have prescribed remain sufficient, so far, to reverse the process. If not, I proceed to the next level—increased steroids—and, if that doesn't work, my last "at home" resort is the epi pen, which I continue to carry with me at all times. Short of that, it's 911.

That being said, I like my sleep. Hiding our electronic Scrabble game under the blankets, in an effort to keep the light from waking Eddie, the computer has the decided advantage at two A.M. while I compete against it in an attempt to keep my heavy eyes from closing. Ironically, on the most painful nights, even the sandman can't win, however. My mind is too pre-occupied with "what ifs".

What if I make a judgement mistake in deciding when I'm in too much trouble to treat tonight's flare myself? What if I don't choose the correct pill? What if the dose I select is too little—or too high? What if I do go to the hospital only to hear doing so was unnecessary? What if I don't go and my family has to live with a morbid mistake I could have prevented? Understandably, these unrelenting "what ifs" that swim through my head on my most physically challenging nights are NOT sleep conducive!

Within twenty minutes of my doctor's resident entering the exam room and questioning me thoroughly, it becomes abundantly clear that I'm not the only person aware that I'm saving my own life—and precariously so. Her questions are not only insightful and thought-provoking, but somewhat scary—in a compassionate way. Inquiring as to whether I always carry an epi pen, when I respond affirmatively she asks if I know how to use it. Assuring her that I do, she surprises me by inquiring that I explain the procedure to her. Though initially dumbfounded by this unexpected request no other physician ever presented, it occurs to me it could be a life-saving one. For example, she shares something I never knew—nor included in my explanation—that it should be administered without holding the top, to avoid injuring the thumb. Further, I'm told it is preferable to inject while lying down rather than sitting up. Her graphic description to hold it "icepick—like" produces a memorable image in my mind—one I hope and suspect, despite challenged clarity in thinking I would invariably assume occurs in emergent situations serious enough to require epi pen usage—I will never forget.

Completing her interview portion of the visit, she ushers us into my doctor's office where she waits with us for her, by-now, predictably welcoming smile, which arrives moments later. Once we are seated, she begins by summarizing their lack of effective results. With all the compassion eyes can reflect, she states the obvious—the desensitizing isn't working in my case. If anything, the reactions worsen with each administration. (Truthfully, after the last one, when the infusion had to be stopped multiple times, so that antihistamines could be dispensed by I.V. to counteract chest tightness, lip tingling, itchiness, etc.,—all indications of an adverse reaction, with the potential to become more serious if not arrested in time—I don't want to chance another dose.)

If eyes could plead, I can almost feel mine doing so as I look directly into hers, silently begging not to hear the words I know are coming next—but I can't avoid. Continuing, as humbly as one can deliver a message—the importance of which I can't afford to miss—she points out that I have been evaluated by the most specialized center for desensitization I can go to. There is no more advanced facility for an immune system as compromised as mine, in terms of achieving successful desensitizing.

My respect for this doctor escalates by the minute when she shares that physicians learn more from their failures than their successes and I've taught them so much by coming to them for treatment. If only every physician realized what it means to a patient to have such an accomplished doctor—from a renowned facility recognized for its successfully high percentage rate in solving cases others could not—admit that their institution "owned" the lack of a cure, (where applicable), rather than devising a way of justifying or sheltering their inability to help every patient. Logically, even the most brilliant medical minds would be unrealistically challenged if expected to cure each patient they see.

Listening to this physician hold herself, her colleagues and their hospital more accountable—in an unapologetic way with each successive word—her explanation professionally echoes what I've just attempted to convey—that no one can expect to have ALL the answers. Impressed with the human side of medicine that she doesn't hesitate to share, I can't help but contrast it to the way others blamed the patient for the medical profession's lack of answers. With labels like "anxiety", and statements such as: "sometimes it only FEELS like throat constriction but really isn't", "swollen lips don't count if they swell down into the face rather than straight out", and several other inane excuses for the inability to diagnose, I can understand why misdiagnosis statistics are so high. At the same time, I'm encouraged to note the difference in the humility demonstrated by my current immunologist. Is there any doubt as to why she is so successful and in demand?

Giving her a hug, it is with the realization that I'm saying good-bye to a physician I don't want to leave—one who is so down to earth and real—at the same time secure to the point she doesn't need to pretend she is infallible. With not a drop of "doctor god" blood flowing through her veins, I could only hope there are enough role models like herself to instruct current medical students.

Too proud to do so in her presence, as we leave her office suite and enter the hallway I know only too well I'll never step foot in again, I no longer will my eyes to hold back the couple of tears begging to trickle down my cheeks—bathing them with regret that the desensitization we'd had such high hopes for failed. Understandably disappointed, generating the tears is the realization that I tried so hard to exhaust every possibility to eradicate these scary and, potentially deadly symptoms—only to be no better off than when this frustrating medical nightmare first began.

CHAPTER THIRTEEN

"The Best Day of Her Life"

"Love everyone in your life for any moment could be their last."

—Anonymous

Advising me that my latest book author luncheon will be held at a beautiful resort close by, the bookseller considerately gives me a choice of several dates, one of which coincidentally falls on my mother's 87th birthday. While I can't explain it—and despite selecting it means that previous plans would prevent people I want to go from attending—I feel a strong and hauntingly incessant nudge to choose mom's birthday. Deciding to go with this silent yet unrelenting message, I schedule it with the intention of surprising her. Calling mom's best friend, who typically takes her out to lunch on her birthday, I share my plan—at the same time requesting that she be an integral part of it by asking her to become my "excuse" for getting her there. As expected because she would do anything for my mom, she enthusiastically agrees. Before getting off, I swear her to secrecy—doing the same with others I call to let in on the surprise.

Upon receiving the excited call I was expecting from my mom, she regurgitates details that I not only already know—but planned. Exuberantly, she relates how she is going to a restaurant on the shore, (at a to-date undisclosed location), that she will be having her hair done before, etc. There is almost a child-like giddiness in her voice—something we've heard before and one of the things we love about her. Listening to her exude such happiness, and at the same time "senior innocence", brings a smile to my heart—one that although I can't see it, I know is inarguable. Every excited detail she shares makes the pitch of her voice get higher. As long as I can remember, she has looked forward to her birthdays with much anticipation—and from what I sense, her approaching one is no exception.

I, too, am excited about the event. I know of approximately fifty people planning to attend, not the least of whom is my daughter, Storey, and her family. This is especially significant because my mom has been longing to meet her youngest great grandchild, Storey's son, who is only months old and lives out of state. The thought of her surprising mom with his presence brings out the child in me. I find myself bursting with close-to-impossible-to-contain enthusiasm, similar to what I felt when surprising my children, years ago, with a trip to Disney World the night before we were to leave. It takes more self-control than I thought I had to bite my tongue and come up with believable answers during the next few months, whenever she asks when she will get to meet her youngest great-grandson.

Ironically, although I absolutely love surprising others, I'm not a person who is easily surprised, generally figuring it out ahead of time—and my daughter Stacey is just like me when it comes to enjoying surprising others. Because I know that, (and her!), I am highly suspicious when a good luck package arrives in the mail just days before the book author luncheon. Filled with all my favorite goodies, it also includes a very touching card with not only her own sentiments, but regrets that she is unable to attend because of a pre-planned trip to Florida on the same day as the talk. However, she wanted me to know they would be thinking of me. As if a light switch turns on in my brain, at that very moment I know she and her family will be traveling the four-and-a-half-hour car ride to surprise me—and I'm touched from head-to-toe with her unspoken, (but no longer clandestine), plan.

Now I have a "mom" dilemma. Do I let on that I know and spoil it for her, or do I play along? Deciding to go with it for the few remaining days, I listen as she describes her family's travel plans, (which I know will occur but not until AFTER the book author luncheon).

With the event planned, I go to my regular hairdresser in preparation. While there, I describe what I'm doing the next day and my excitement over surprising my mom. Before I can finish, I'm stunned speechless by what happens next. Have you ever experienced seeing someone you know, at a distance, but in a different way than you are accustomed to seeing them—perhaps in a way you would prefer not to admit visualizing them? A frail, older-looking thin woman, dependent upon a cane, enters the salon—oblivious of me as it takes all her concentration to navigate to a seat. I can feel the hair stand up on my arms at the realization that the woman is my mom—however, not the vibrant one I've known all these years; instead, one that has aged before my disbelieving eyes, in a way until now, I refused to see—or didn't want to. It is almost like I am looking at a person I don't know, whose seemingly overnight transformation raises concerns about the mortality of someone I always, unrealistic as it may be, thought would live forever.

Involuntarily stiffening as my eyes brim with unshed tears, my hairdresser picks up on my out-of-character body language, inquiring with undisguised concern as to what is wrong. In a subdued, I-can't-believe-this-is-happening, somewhat shocked voice, I explain that the lady who just walked in, the one the staff readily offers to physically assist, is my mom. Ironically, neither she nor I realized we went to the same salon.

Swearing my hairdresser to secrecy regarding tomorrow's event, I impulsively walk toward my mom, who is approaching her own hair stylist, wondering how long it will take before she notices me.

Her surprised look is only matched by the one that transformed my face when she first walked in. Bending over to kiss her cheek, she tells me she is having her hair done because of her birthday luncheon tomorrow. After discussing the irony of us both going to the same salon for many years, while unbeknown to either of us, we then exchange a few minutes of further small talk. Anxious to leave before I accidentally let the cat out of the bag, I wish her a nice time with her friend, promising we'll get together later in the weekend to celebrate.

Arriving home, I decide the "secret" with Stacey has outlived its practicality. I know she and her entire family, including our son-in-law and four of our six grandchildren, are in a nearby hotel. Since we only get to see each other every six weeks or so, given they live such a distance away, do I really intend to miss the opportunity to spend time with them tonight? No way!

"Okay, Stace, I guess we are too much alike for me not to be onto you. As much as I appreciate the surprise efforts you made toward tomorrow's book author luncheon, I happen to know you guys are just minutes away—so where are we going for dinner?" Laughing, she tells me that they had every intention of spending this time with us and, within a few minutes our house is filled with the happy chaos of loved ones who've missed each other, excitedly competing for their spot in "catch-up" conversation.

Arriving early at the beautiful resort where the book author luncheon will be held, I'm particularly pleased to see that the room reserved is one with the ocean as a backdrop. Looking in, a wedding could be held here, with linen table décor, sparkling silver utensils and crystal glasses from which one can see the ocean's reflection. The glistening sun adds warmth to the room's already bright and charming window-lined architecture. Having had the opportunity to familiarize myself with my soon-to-be-speaking-at podium, I'm then ushered out so that I can be "introduced" after all the guests have arrived and are seated.

Climbing the plush, floral carpeted stairway to the chandeliered, tastefully-decorated large main lobby, I'm once again taken a little aback when I spot my mom at a distance. She is seated on an upholstered side chair, adjacent to the main door of the resort. With the circular drive-way immediately behind her, I surmise her friend must have dropped her off while she went to park the car—a smart move given how frail she looks to me. Then again, she's lost over fifty pounds in the past year. Am I being too critical, my wishful-thinking brain cells ask?

Approaching her, I'm faced with another concern. While it could be the unexpected surprise of seeing me—and my picture on the main lobby easel, announcing the book author luncheon—(which I want to believe), even strong denial refuses to keep me from observing an uncharacteristic, sort of disoriented demeanor that I'm unaccustomed to seeing in her. Whether overwhelmed from what she hadn't predicted, I can't say—but it scares me.

The arrival of more guests temporarily distracts me from

thoughts I'd rather not face. Everyone is directed to the room where the talk is scheduled to occur. I suppose I should feel nervous at the moment, given the number of people who come up to me and ask if I am, but the truth is I'm not. I know my topic well because I live it—firsthand. Instead of feeling anxious, I look at this as an opportunity to educate others—not only regarding Behcet's, but rare diseases in general. If what I share can prevent one patient from losing their eyesight and/or their life, it will be time well invested.

Before I start, a scrumptious lunch is served, though eating is the last thing on my mind. Instead, I migrate from table to table, mingling with my guests. Despite how involved I am once the talk begins, there are intense, compassionate reactions in the wall-to-wall crowded room that do not escape my notice. For example, my mom repeatedly dabbing her tears during descriptive incidents that are difficult for her to learn I endured. On the positive side, pride reflects back at me from the faces of devoted family and friends.

Truthfully, I can't remember when I've been in a room surrounded by more loving and healing messages telepathically being sent my way—and it feels good.

Following the talk, cake is served, accompanied by more than fifty voices singing Happy Birthday to my mom. Sitting at a small sweetheart table stacked with books to autograph, I'm vaguely aware of a silent but awed presence. Looking to my left, positioned between me and the line of guests patiently waiting for their books to be signed, (holding back a little as though he doesn't know if it is okay to approach the table), I see wide eyes bulging in disbelief, followed by the sentiment, "Pa-Pa, I didn't know that you were famous!" Seconds later, his younger brother, who is eleven, asks, "Pa- Pa, how long have you been famous?" putting into perspective for me that—untrue as that adjective may be—through the eyes of innocent and adoring grandchildren, at this very moment, I guess they think I am—and the pride reflected in their eyes makes my heart smile.

At this point, my mom is in great-grandchild Heaven. Every one of them is engulfing her in quality time and unrelenting love. The photographer positions herself in an attempt to capture my mother with her great-granddaughter sitting on her lap, as my mom holds the back of her head while she and the five-year-old, (obviously younger than described earlier in this book), face each other, lovingly locking eyes. I can only hope this precious-beyond-words pose comes out. It will be like being able to see inside both hearts through the lens of a camera. Why is it I get the feeling that photo will be priceless to people someday missing my mom? Why is it that I fear "someday" is closer than any of us expect?

Was divine intervention responsible for the nudge that directed me to choose my mom's birthday for the speaking event? Could this be the last one we have the opportunity to celebrate, I worry—but pray not?

Fast-forward two and a half months: BLUE LIGHT REFLECTIONS

Bracing myself to explain a decision my heart told me was the only one to make, I transform my face from sadness I refuse to show, to a convincing smile—one that is plastic only to me. Tenderly placing my mom's frail, weak hand into my own, (as my mind asks itself in somewhat disbelief, or more accurately, denial—how this dynamic woman has aged to this point, seemingly overnight), I will my ready-to-spill tears not to dare.

Instead, in a voice that exudes far more acceptance of the idea than I feel, given the finality I associate with admittance to Hospice, I nonchalantly tell her that she is being moved to another floor. Unwilling to allow her mind time to formulate the understandable questions I anticipate, I distract her thought process in another direction, focusing on everything but the real reason for the move. As expected, she reacts positively to my description of the private, warmly-decorated, wallpapered rooms on the floor facilitated by a competent, friendly and compassionate staff. Disconcertingly, my false enthusiasm is not enough to convince me. Consequently, it is with considerable trepidation that I accompany mom to the Hospice floor.

Yet, to my relief, when the elevator door opens, I immediately sense an all-encompassing, overwhelming peacefulness I hadn't noticed anywhere else in the entire facility. While intellectually there is no disputing we are in a hospital, it is easy to momentarily forget. Though I can't pinpoint any one thing that makes me feel this way, I suspect the soft, soothing music as we walk through hallways wafting with the aroma of freshly baking brownies doesn't hurt. In addition, the sterility, though present, is camouflaged with wooden furniture replacing the usual metal institutional pieces. Unable to resist the urge to peek into the rooms we pass, each successive one seems more "homey" and inviting. We pass cozy sitting areas with upholstered chairs, soft lights and filled bookcases; in addition, a community kitchen, a chapel and much more. It is like these corridors reach out and hug everyone who passes through them—at a time when patients and families need them most—and it feels good. Silently, I say a prayer that my mom will be in good hands.

Little can I predict, as I admire the comfy, hand-stitched quilts on each bed, that during some of my most challenging days sitting at my mom's bedside, watching her sleep as I unsuccessfully try to compartmentalize the inevitable, while selfishly prolonging the present, that the day will come when I long for someone to wrap one of these cozy quilts around me—and make it "all better". Instead, my "quilt" is emotional, coming in the form of tender words, touches and gestures from a compassionate and perceptive staff. Whether offering a cup of coffee, a more comfortable chair or a gentle reminder that I have to eat, too, Hospice extends its patient care to include the entire family.

Most importantly, my mom receives impeccable care. In addition to obvious medical competency, her day nurse demonstrates incredible perception and love in the way she treats her. She always has a smile on her face, accompanied by kind, caring words that reflect understanding of the situation. She has a gift of making even awkward situations less so. Independent as my mom was, it is difficult for her to allow others to assist her now that she is unable to feed herself. Wrapping her arms around her, her nurse kindly explains to her that everyone needs a little help sometime, causing my mom to look up at her with appreciation as she cooperatively opens her mouth to accept the spoonful of food she offers.

When my mom becomes ill to the point that her color begins to leave her—something I mention with unmistakable concern in my voice—her nurse changes her pillowcase from white to lavender, to match the pretty nightgown she'd selected for her earlier that day, purposely minimizing the effects of her worsening state. While I have no doubt that this thoughtful gesture is more for my benefit than that of my mom, it is the little things that count at times like this—and her nurse knows just what we need.

Then, just before the angels call my mom, one calls me—in the form of her night nurse, who respected my previously charted request to be notified of any changes, regardless of the hour. With the phone ringing at 1:45 A.M. leaving little to the imagination, a tight knot forms in my stomach as I answer it, expecting to hear she has passed. Instead, a kind but concerned voice on the other end explains she has been my mom's middle of the night nurse during the past week and for the first time she is detecting a noticeable change in her breathing. Informing her that it is my intent to come to the hospital, (reminding her that I live a half hour away), I ask her to call me in the meantime should she think that isn't a good idea. My unspoken message, which I can't bring myself to verbalize, but she gets loud and clear, is that if she should pass.

Two minutes after we hang up, the phone rings again. This time, the same nurse delivers a far more significant message. With gentleness and compassion, I am tenderly informed that my mom is very close to taking her last breath. Making a decision the impact of which I can't begin to know at the time, she says she is putting the phone to her ear so I can speak to her, which I do for a minute or two. While one might wonder how much could be said in such a short period of time, I have no trouble finding the words I need and want to say—words that are compassionately interrupted by the nurse informing me that she has her stethoscope and is listening, knowing she is close. Seconds later, she tells me my mom has "left us". Even as tears stream down my face, I somehow have the presence of mind to croak out a thank you for a gift I will forever hold in my heart—sharing my mom's last minutes with her.

For the rest of my life, I will thank God that I chose mom's birthday for my surprise book author luncheon. Describing it as "the best day of her life", those are words I will never forget.

***

Unfortunately, we are at the ages when, statistically,

most of our parents pass—and our family is no exception. Consequently, though expectedly sad it comes as no surprise when losses happen in close succession—but it doesn't make it any easier.

On August 2, within hours of being comforted by her 20-month old youngest great-grandchild, singing his tender version of "Twinkle, Twinkle, Little Star" to "Grammy" while lovingly blowing kisses at her bedside, Eddie's mom passed peacefully at her home. Whether it was the innocence of a child's angelic voice that allowed her a preview of Heaven—causing her to pursue entrance—we can only speculate. Though too young to remember those special final moments he spent with this remarkable woman during her last hours, we're not. It is an image that will forever warm our hearts—and a story we will share with her youngest great-grandson when he is old enough to understand. May God Bless you, Grammy!

CHAPTER FOURTEEN

Disconcerting Statistics

"Mistakes are lessons inside out." —Matshona Dhliwayo

While it is human nature to become defensive about errors made in occupations we trained long and hard to achieve proficiency in, the reality is mistakes happen. However, when they impact life and death, inarguably serious action must be taken to address them. Consequently, it comes as no surprise that the media has dedicated so much air time and ink to publicizing the unacceptably high statistics associated with medical errors. In response, the medical community reacted to the disconcertingly undeniable numbers, by publicly recognizing the need for aggressive action through concerted efforts—in recent years—to reduce and/or eradicate medical mistakes. Understandably, changes to the extent these statistics associated with misdiagnosis require, do not occur overnight. Rather, it is a process—a necessary one which will undoubtedly educate current and prospective physicians, not only by providing an awareness of past errors so that they are not repeated, but by creating innovative programs to anticipate and prevent them—hopefully resulting in life-saving treatment for patients they now administer care to—and those in the future.

To justify recent concern over misdiagnosis, and in an attempt to put it in perspective, I first researched several studies and authors addressing the magnitude of the problem. After compiling statistics and specific examples of mistakes reported by the media, (undoubtedly scaring the general public—and understandably so), I then investigated efforts that have been initiated and/or are currently being instituted by the medical profession to address and significantly lower these unacceptable numbers. Following is a sample of what my research uncovered:

Inaccurate diagnosis, a much more clandestine topic in the past, (in part due to physicians' reluctance to share such information because of unfortunate, but at times, realistic concerns over potential punitive repercussions and/or peer disrespect), has been disclosed like never before. The fact that an international conference on misdiagnosis occurred, in which the problem was shared objectively, is a reflection of this. "Misdiagnosis happens all the time", according to David Newman-Toker, M.D., PhD, and organizer of the conference. He and his colleague, Peter Pronovost, M.D., PhD., authored "Diagnostic Errors—Next Frontier for Patient Safety", which was published in the "Journal of the American Medical Association", (JAMA). In it, they disclosed previously unshared information with lay people regarding the number of hospital deaths in the United States, yearly, due to misdiagnosis. According to one media report, it has been said that this "groundbreaking article" "Blew the lid off this scandal". (My personal interpretation was that rather than a "scandal", it was a serious situation that required immediate and aggressive intervention.) Though the doctors initially reported the number of deaths to be between 40,000 and 80,000, a subsequent radio interview with them indicated that these numbers were conservative. Disconcertingly, the amount of deaths was more accurately about 100,000.

According to The Institute of Medicine, (I.O.M.), a worldwide organization noted for its expertise on the subject, their objective statistics indicate that misdiagnosis is attributable to 10% of patient deaths, resulting in diagnostic mistakes rating as the third leading cause of death in the U.S. In "Alternative Diagnosis", a report by CNN, surveys corroborated this finding with the probability of misdiagnosis falling between 8 and 40%, proving it to be one of the most prevalent medical mistakes. According to I.O.M. statistics, over 18 million errors, by primary care providers, are made yearly in the U.S.

In "Misdiagnosis: A Big Problem"—All Too Common Errors Have Deadly Potential, (The Hartford Courant, 5-19-13), Christine Cassel, a participant on the panel responsible for composing the 1999 IOM report, To Err is Human: Building a Safer Health System, (a comprehensive approach to eliminate as many preventable medical mistakes as possible)—and subsequent President and Chief Executive Officer of the American Board of Internal Medicine—makes the interesting observation and, in my opinion, potentially life-saving point that, despite the number of quality measures we now use in assuming that a diagnosis is the right one, what if it isn't?

Dr. Graber, (President of the Society to Improve Diagnosis in Medicine), provides a graphic analogy when he compares the E.R. to a "petri dish" for diagnostic mistakes. Considering the combination of physicians unfamiliar with patients they are probably seeing for the first time, stressed doctors with workloads they can't do justice to, patients who don't know them—and, therefore, haven't established trust in, his point is well taken.

I especially appreciate his objectivity when he open-mindedly shares, "Overconfidence in our abilities is part of the problem. Physicians don't know how error-prone they are". He feels that doctors have been allowed a "pass" when it comes to diagnostic accuracy—for too extended a period of time.

From firsthand experience and subsequent research, I respect his point, which I believe many of the following specific misdiagnoses cases are evidence of.

In her article, "Could You Have Been Misdiagnosed?", by Brenda Goodman, staff writer for WebMD, she describes a patient who was diagnosed by a neurologist as having carpal tunnel syndrome. Her internist said it was the flu. Having been mislabeled by thirteen previous physicians, an orthopedic surgeon finally confirmed, by x-ray, the accurate diagnosis: rheumatoid arthritis.

***

According to "Why Doctors So Often Get It Wrong", by David Leonhardt, New York Times, Business Daily, (February, 2006), studies of autopsy reports indicate that doctors misdiagnose illnesses—at times life-threateningly—approximately 20% of the time. The ramifications of this statistic are that millions of patients are receiving inappropriate treatment because of an incorrectly diagnosed condition. Even more disconcerting, according to the article, is that things really haven't changed enough to affect improvement since the 1930's. Leonhardt refers to a Journal of American Medical Association publication which straight-forwardly acknowledges the problem as: No Improvement! From my interpretation of Leonhardt's newspaper report, despite the impressive amount of money the U.S., (the wealthiest country in the world), devotes to healthcare, not enough is allocated specifically to misdiagnosis.

One point the author makes, which the idealistic part of me wants to believe is not true, (and that compassion would overrule this in the way they practice), is that because medical personnel are less financially reimbursed for determining the correct diagnosis than to execute tests, perform surgery and give out drugs—there is less appeal to expend as much time and effort on rarer, atypical presenting conditions. Couldn't that, alone, be responsible for inflated misdiagnoses rates? And, if so, how many patients do we have to lose before we prioritize differently? Further, what will it take to ensure procedures for cross-checking diagnoses are in place?

Joseph Britto, (former intensive care doctor), presents a perspective that, in my mind, says it all. When comparing medical errors to those incurred by airlines, he notes how pilots, by insisting that all errors be investigated, (because THEIR lives were on the line), successfully eradicated the majority of potential crashes. "Unlike pilots, Dr. Britto perceptively points out, "doctors don't go down with their planes."

* * *

Reporter Jamie Docherme, in "Misdiagnosing Cancer is More Common Than We Think", (HOB Health, January 31, 2013), shares that "Best Doctors, Inc." found cancer is commonly misdiagnosed. Interestingly, though, a study conducted between Best Doctors and The National Coalition on Health Care revealed 60.5% of doctors questioned estimated cancer misdiagnosis rates to be zero to 10%, in decided contrast to the British Medical Journal (BMJ) Quality and Safety Journal which believes it to be closer to 28%.

When asked if misdiagnosis is the result of doctors who don't care—or aren't committed, David Seligman, Chairman and Chief Executive Officer of Best Doctors, unhesitatingly responds, "Of course not,", "But doctors today are increasingly time-strapped. Many of them are seeing up to 30 patients a day. They're working in an overburdened health system with fractured or incomplete medical records. All of these things too often directly impact health outcomes—no matter how dedicated or skilled the physician may be."

According to Thomson Reuters, "Nearly seven hundred billion dollars are wasted in the U.S. medical system each year, much of which is tied to misdiagnosis or people getting the wrong treatment." John Rother, National Coalition on Healthcare, (NCHC), President and Chief Executive Officer, believes, "Not enough is being done on the state and federal policy end of things to acknowledge and firmly address this critical issue. Given our current health care climate and challenges, as decision-makers become more aware of the frequency of misdiagnosis and the enormous costs associated with it, they have a sizeable opportunity to make diagnostic accuracy much more of a 'front and center' issue in health care."

***

According to Ashley Strickland, in her CNN broadcast on Monday, August 1, 2016, a 23-year old Master's Degree Candidate who worked in the health field was in intense stomach pain—so severe that she was eventually diagnosed with Crohn's. However, logistically this explanation was not valid given her blood counts subsequently did not recover with treatment.

Convinced something worse was going on, she scheduled a bone marrow biopsy, which elucidated the diagnosis of myeloid leukemia, a rare, aggressive blood cancer. Because this type of cancer can kill within six weeks without treatment, according to this medically trained patient, she was immediately started on chemotherapy and subsequently successfully underwent a bone marrow transplant.

"I cannot emphasize how important it is to advocate for yourself in our health care system," said patient Leeanne Hester. "I didn't shy away from asking questions and pushing for answers, because I knew something wasn't right with my body. I even had to call and remind one of my specialists that I needed to schedule a follow-up appointment. Had I waited even a month or two, it may have been too late."

In my opinion, in addition to her medical background, she owes the fact that she is alive to tell her story to her persistence in insisting that something was wrong—and not giving up until she was heard and appropriately treated.

***

In "Chronic Neuro Immune Disease" by Michelle Bloomquish, Web M.D., Medical News, January 1, 2014, she describes how many autoimmune diseases such as lupus, scleroderma and rheumatoid arthritis are frequently misdiagnosed, (a reality I, like so many others, lived firsthand). Many years ago, actress Kellie Martin's sister, 19 at the time, presented with baffling symptoms including fatigue, an unusual skin rash and a multitude of other medical abnormalities. Despite the variety of diagnoses her doctors labeled her with—and, in some cases attempts utilizing various treatments—she continued to become more seriously ill. Inexplicably weaker and weaker, she was eventually diagnosed correctly—with systemic lupus erythematosus.

Autoimmune diseases such as hers are characterized by immune systems that go into overdrive. Not only do they attack unwanted foreign invaders, but they also mistake the body's necessary vital organs as those that need to be destroyed as well.

According to the article, these diseases affect 50 million Americans, 75% of whom are women, (as stated by Virginia Ladd, president and founder of The American Autoimmune Related Diseases Association, Inc.—and a lupus patient, herself). Frustratingly, there is no one specialist to consult for these diseases. Instead, patients go to doctors based on the symptoms they exhibit. For example, someone with skin rashes may see a dermatologist, while patients challenged by bone pain may go to a rheumatologist, and so forth. Ladd makes a meaningful analogy when she states "It is like trying to fight cancer, but with no oncologist". It is Ladd's hope that a new specialty, where patients presenting with these diseases could schedule with an "auto immunologist", will be developed in the near future. (I, too, would like to see this development. Patients with autoimmune diseases are often far too ill to travel from one specialist to the next seeking a diagnosis for the various seemingly-unrelated symptoms they present with. Having a physician knowledgeable in making the connection would ease their diagnostic process tremendously, allowing them to use their compromised energy more efficiently. What I would have given to have had an "auto immunologist" to consult when my disease first manifested!)

Another female patient, Linda Otto, realized firsthand the difficulty in obtaining a diagnosis for strange symptoms that stumped her physicians—and the battle she had to fight to get an explanation when her doctors couldn't provide one. While unsuccessfully pursuing an answer, Linda says, "I was terrified. I thought I was going to die. Nobody could tell me about the disease, what to expect or how to treat it." Like me, she traveled cross-country, desperately seeking a diagnosis.

It was during filming of a documentary with Bob Saget that she was overcome by serious symptoms no one could explain. Reaching out to her with the compassion of someone who understood her frustration firsthand, he shared that his sister was dying of scleroderma, (an autoimmune disease that involves hardening of the connective tissues in the skin). Ironically, Linda was diagnosed with the same illness the day after Bob's sister's funeral.

Over the past several decades I've had the opportunity to speak at joint meetings for lupus and scleroderma patients. My recollection of many of the scleroderma patients I encountered is that they exhibited a characteristic "tightness" in their smiles—almost unnaturally wrinkle-free looking, with a sense of permanence that never seems to go away.

While this kind of stiffening can be detected by the casual, non-medically-trained observer, it is the type the article describes that we cannot see, (but attacks crucial organs, with potentially deadly ramifications)—that concerns me more. When vital organs like the lungs are involved, functioning is challenged and/or prevented.

Despite grim predictions dispensed by her physicians that she never would, Linda was able to achieve full use of her hands, (through alternative medicine)—including disproving that they would clench beyond the ability to function. According to the author, Ladd, Otto and Martin, (and, from my firsthand perspective, Eileen Radziunas!), all encourage women to pursue other diagnoses if they think something is physically wrong, regardless if subsequent to having been told nothing was. Frustratingly, accurate diagnosis of an autoimmune disease may require consulting multiple physicians, sometimes over a period of months and/or years. Ladd echoes my sentiments when she states, "You have to keep believing in yourself, even if everyone is saying it's all in your head". "Don't give up until you get a diagnosis."

Her words send a river of reality through my veins, chilling them from head-to-toe. If only there was an eraser strong enough to eradicate the horrific memory of those pre-diagnostic years of feeling sicker than I've ever been in my entire life—only to be told "It's all in your head", by physicians too inexperienced with the presentation of my atypical symptoms to accurately diagnose them. Searching the thesaurus of my mind, I come up empty looking for a word powerful enough to describe how that hurt—more importantly, how much premature dismissal such as that not only inflates misdiagnosis statistics but, can result in life-threatening ramifications.

While aware the entire time of those who doubted the authenticity of a real physical illness, (sentiments like that have a way of seeping out), it was even more disconcerting to learn that their misjudgments had been shared with others.

However, challenging as it might have been, (and make no mistake, it was!), through it all I was determined to stay true to myself as I had no doubt my life depended on it. No one knew this body like the person encased in it—and something was clearly abnormal. If it took more than 100 physicians to solve my medical mystery, which it eventually did, I had no intention of giving up. There was an answer out there and I owed it to myself and my family to find it. Interestingly, once I did several people asked me if at any time before receiving it I questioned whether something was really going on, physically. Each time, my answer was an emphatic "No!". Kellie Martin verbalized a disconcerting reality most of us can relate to when she said, "Often the biggest obstacle that patients with autoimmune disease face is just getting a diagnosis". From firsthand experience, I would add that even with one, the most many autoimmune patients can expect, based on current medical knowledge, is symptomatic treatment—until further research is done. Noel R. Rose, professor of pathology and immunology at Johns Hopkins University in Baltimore echoes this disappointing reality when he explains that while they are aggressively trying to find a trigger for these diseases, until they do there is no cure—only treatment for the symptoms. In the meantime, he, like Ladd, Otto, Martin and myself, recommends that despite being told nothing is wrong at past evaluations, if a patient still feels physically ill they should pursue additional consultations.

It saddens me to report that soon after getting her diagnosis, Kellie's sister Heather died of a lung infection which challenged her immune system beyond its capabilities, considering the stress it was already under. Kellie's contention—and I tend to agree with her—is that an earlier diagnosis could have saved her life. "If a doctor dismisses symptoms or says they are stress-related, patients need to find another doctor—period", she says. (With sincerest thanks to Kellie Martin for going public with her sister's story so that others will benefit—and to Bob Saget for helping autoimmune patients everywhere through his sister's story. Know that each of you have my sincerest condolences regarding the loss of your loved ones.)

***

In "When Your Doctor Mislabels You as an Anxious Female", by Carolyn Thomas, (Heart Sisters, June 4, 2016), she states: "Take it from me, the only thing worse than a heart attack is being misdiagnosed and sent home from the hospital while you're having it. And for women in particular this is a tragically all-too-common reality."

The New England Journal of Medicine researched misdiagnosed cardiac cases, reviewing 10,000. Almost half, (48%), were women. Each patient had gone to their emergency departments due to noteworthy chest pain and/or other heart attack indications. According to the study, women younger than 55 were 7 times more likely to be sent home than males, regardless of presenting with equally severe symptoms. (I must admit, as a woman with heart issues—despite the fact that I'm older than 55—this makes me feel very insecure!)

The results reported that women dismissed during heart attacks had double the chance of dying. Those patients fortunate enough to live to tell about heart attacks they experienced shared the misdiagnoses they were given, some of which included: indigestion, stress, pulled muscles, gall bladder, etc. But one of the most dismissive misdiagnoses to "drip from the lips of an emergency department physician is ANXIETY". It is my interpretation from what I read, that this psychiatric stereotype generates unnecessary, unrelated testing which the patient must endure—despite being so physically ill—unless her cardiac investigation shows measurable, potentially fatal heart attack suspicion.

Cornell University conducted a study entitled "Gender Bias in the Diagnosis, Treatment and Interpretation of Coronary Heart Disease Symptoms". The results, which were published in 2008, were disconcerting. At a scientific cardio-vascular research foundation meeting, symptoms were compared with the intent of deciding whether female patients exhibiting similar ones were handled differently, based on their sex.

Disturbingly, the results indicated less women were likely to receive a coronary heart disease diagnosis when stress was implied. The figures showed that when symptoms were similar, 30% of women were referred to cardiology, while 62% of men were. Additionally, heart medications were prescribed less often for women, (13%), as compared to men, (47%). Not only is this information frustrating—but, more importantly, dangerous. I find it unconscionable that the same symptoms in a woman, such as chest pain, shortness of breath, irregular heartbeat, etc., can be labeled stress—but cardiac in a male. (Hmm, one would think not being taken seriously enough with those symptoms, and/or being dismissed with a less life-threatening label—while accurately fearing she is the only one aware of the gravity of the situation—might be a stressor in itself!)

According to Alexandra J. Lansky, Director of the Women's Health Initiative at the Cardiovascular Research Foundation, "We know there is a delay in diagnosing coronary heart disease in women and this study is an important step forward in understanding why."

***

In "How Doctors Think", two of the most respected researchers studying medical communication share their thoughts—ones I feel could influence and lessen misdiagnosis statistics if respected. Debra Roter, Professor of Health Policy and Management at Johns Hopkins University and Judith Hall, a Professor of Social Psychology at Northeastern University have reviewed thousands of patient videotapes—in addition to live conversations. Their research indisputably demonstrated the necessity for a patient to feel free to share their thoughts and emotions, providing important diagnostic clues. I couldn't agree more with Hall's observation, "If a patient is inhibited, or cut off prematurely, or constrained into one path of discussion then the doctor may not be told something vital". According to her, doctors interrupt their patients within eighteen seconds of them beginning to speak. (While I've experienced inconsideration such as this in the past, on the positive side, it is certainly NOT exhibited by the specialists I currently see—which, because they listen intently to what I have to say, is probably why I am accurately diagnosed and under appropriate protocol for my conditions.) Another observation Hall made that I can really relate to is that the sickest patients are, at times, the ones physicians like least—(a reality perceptive patients are well aware of from the way they are treated). According to her, when this occurs it is initiated by the doctors' own frustrations in being unable to make a positive difference despite their best efforts. Because of that, they give up. (To me, personally, I equate examples of this as being told—angrily—to find a new doctor, that I have too many symptoms, that I'm wasting their time when I don't need them and other patients do, etc.) While I understand projection of one's frustrations onto another, in my opinion patients with life-threatening conditions require and deserve much better than this.

I think Dr. Jerome Groopman makes an important distinction between medical mistakes and misdiagnosis in his book, "How Doctors Think". He contends: "Medical mistakes have been written about extensively in the lay press and analyzed in a report from the Institute of Medicine of the National Academy of Sciences. They involve prescribing the wrong dose of a drug or looking at an x-ray of a patient backward. Misdiagnosis is different. It is a window into the medical mind. It reveals why doctors fail to question their medical assumptions, why their thinking is sometimes closed or skewed, why they overlook the gaps in their knowledge. Experts studying misguided care have recently concluded that the majority of errors are due to flaws in physician thinking, not technical mistakes." One of the studies he utilized for this information was a 1995 report citing that up to 15% of all diagnoses are inaccurate, in which doctors reviewed written descriptions of patients' symptoms and examined patient-actors emulating a variety of diseases.

Dr. Groopman contends that doctors' inner feelings are responsible for cognitive errors in practicing medicine—emotions they are reluctant to admit and/or are unaware of.

I found it educational but at the same time disconcerting, to read his section referring to "confirmation bias", a concept he explains as, (in my layman's terms of interpretation), labeling what you expect to find by selectively weeding out or not incorporating all the information presented. This close-minded approach leaves no room for other disease considerations—(particularly rare ones with less easily identifiable symptoms)—and, as far as I'm concerned, enables misdiagnosis.

It brought tears to my eyes to read his account of a woman referred to a psychiatrist because of her "psychosomatic" pain—and that a triage nurse, upon hearing she was back after previously being worked up, rolled her eyes at her in disgust. It took repeated, tearful visits, (trust me, I'd be at another facility by then!), with the patient insisting no one believed her, before her ruptured ectopic pregnancy was discovered. (Why is it as I type this my husband's words—words he used repeatedly through my medical mysteries, resound with haunting, but at the same time inarguable truth:" Healthy until proven ill"?) What else could this woman have done to demonstrate how sick she really was? To think she was demeaned while desperately making her best attempts to be heard—as she endured unbearable, dismissed pain—is unconscionable.

* * *

If any misdiagnosis story hugged my heart in an unforgettable way, it was one described in an article by Melissa McGlensey. In "This Woman Spent Decades Unable to Control Her Limbs—Then One Day Everything Changed", Melissa, who writes for "The Mighty", had this incredible story published in their April 2, 2015 issue.

Relating the account of Jean Sharon Abbott's amazing—yet preventable—medical history, she describes the devastatingly inexcusable predicament of a patient who was debilitated for more than 30 years, barely able to move any appendages, and requiring help with everyday responsibilities most of us do automatically—with no thought involved. But incredulously, one day her world changed.

Though diagnosed at four years old with a condition known as spastic dysplasia, a type of cerebral palsy, none of her MRI's or CAT scans confirmed it. Despite no clinical findings on these tests, her neurologist—one of the best in this specialty—felt her symptoms were classic. At times she sought additional opinions, only to be told by doctors impressed when given the name of the physician who diagnosed her, that he was one of the top.

Consequently, with no other diagnoses assigned, she adjusted her lifestyle to live as productively as possible with her disabilities. She went to school close to home, made friends and cultivated hobbies.

At the age of twelve an operation was performed in an attempt to allow her to walk more comfortably. It involved detaching muscles from her hips and attaching them to her knees— the goal being that they wouldn't hit each other when she tried to walk. Because of this surgery, a full body cast was required for a month, yet, disconcertingly, she appreciated only a slightly improved gait as a result of the operation.

Another procedure was performed in her late twenties, during which a medication dispensing pump was installed, after which a complication resulted in her becoming over medicated. Because of this, she consulted a doctor she hadn't seen before—one who specialized in this equipment.

Unconvinced that she had cerebral palsy, this physician influenced her to seek the opinion of another neurologist. After taking her history, the doctor she was referred to smiled and said, "I think you have Dopa-Responsive Dystonia." (According to the article, this condition, which presents with involuntary muscle contractions and tremors, is often mistaken for other disorders— cerebral palsy being one of them. Actually, its name comes from its positive reaction to the medication L-Dopa.)

Her new neurologist explained that the debilitating symptoms that controlled most of her life—the spasticity, cramping muscles, weakness, etc., would disappear with just a simple pill.

Thinking he must be out of his mind, she told "The Mighty" she initially had no intention of filling the prescription—but did so to appease her husband.

Three hours after ingesting her first dose, she felt slightly stronger. Confirming this was her newfound ability to get up from a chair without help. Incredulously, the next day—after not being able to do so, independently, for a decade—she could stand on her own. It was then that she knew the drugs were working—and that her life had changed, in a most positive way—FOREVER.

* * *

Reading about a stroke patient, (by Kate Davies, "Designs", 2-25-15), who was initially misdiagnosed, resurrected a firsthand nightmare—from a deep, scary place within me that I try not to re-visit—but will, (later in this chapter), for the purpose of lending credibility to the experience of the patient described—by confirming that she is not alone. Suffice it to say at this point, unlike most nightmares which one wakes up from with a sigh of relief, my reality is that I never emitted that sigh—nor felt relief. Now, back to the article from "Designs":

Despite presenting with a droopy face, the inability to go to the bathroom by herself, visual abnormalities, piercing pins-and-needles, difficulty hearing and talking, etc., the patient featured in this account was not admitted to the stroke floor. Fortunately, an astute medical student subsequently examined her and detected that she had a leg that was hyper-reflexive. Suspecting a stroke, she ordered an M.R.I. which, unlike her initial C.A.T. scan, confirmed it.

A blood thinner commonly used to dissolve clots in stroke patients was immediately administered. After multiple additional neurological exams, not only by physicians she had never seen before, but also the neurologist who originally misdiagnosed her, she noticed the staff treated her differently. Compassion and empathy replaced the less concerned demeanors she was originally subjected to before the stroke was recognized. Her needs were now immediately met in a non-dismissive way she wasn't, to this point, accustomed to.

Analyzing this dramatic change in care within one day, she realized that clinical evidence proved she no longer was the hysterical patient she was labeled upon admission; instead, one whose serious stroke had been misdiagnosed and consequently, unaddressed with the degree of concern it demanded.

Though I was once that undiagnosed stroke patient—with stabbing pins-and-needles, leg weakness, swallowing so difficult that I had to sleep sitting up straight for three months, urinary incontinence, etc., unlike her, I felt, (and was), dismissed by the medical profession for far longer—as though I had nothing serious going on. As you know from the beginning of this book, it took more than a decade before my brainstem stroke was diagnosed. Ironically, over twenty years later, when I had a brain bleed, (the effects of which impacted my life considerably less than the first stroke), I was immediately ambulanced to a major stroke center where I was admitted to Neuro-ICU. In contrast to my initial brain infarct, I was almost " coddled" by the attentive staff. My one-on-one nursing care was more dedicated than I can find words to describe. What I would have done to have had that professional support and assistance following my unidentified brain stem stroke! To paraphrase the words of a patient already quoted in this book which stated, "Take it from me, the only thing worse than a heart attack is being misdiagnosed and sent home from the hospital while you're having it", (from the blog in "Heart Sisters", "When Your Doctor Mislabels You an Anxious Female", by Carolyn Thomas), I say "The only thing worse than a brain stem stroke is being misdiagnosed and sent home from the hospital told you hadn't had one—when you had". No patient should ever have to manage such serious symptoms without medical intervention—which, years later, I was informed screamed for rehabilitation that, in my specific case required speech, physical and occupational therapy, and urology studies—at the very least.

Like water in an old-fashioned aluminum coffee pot beginning to simmer when I was a child—before it was quite hot enough to reach and color its clear glass bubble on the lid, but noisily preparing to perk, I sense the effervescence of my blood about to boil. Traversing my veins at what seems like a much faster speed than usual, the difference is that unlike the coffee pot, with its hissing and spitting sounds anyone in earshot can hear, the sensation I experience is silent and internal—but, none-the-less real to me. My face flushing hotter by the minute, I listen attentively to a patient directly across from me, detailing a horrific misdiagnosis account.

"It's all in your head", the desperately ill patient was told. There was talk of admission to the psychiatric wing, a threat her devoted and loving spouse adamantly advocated against. Staring into her gorgeous, intense blue, quarter-sized eyes, she is beautiful even without hair to frame the face that owns them. Its temporary absence, she self-consciously explains, is the result of recent neuro surgery. According to the patient, she was rushed by ambulance from home to a facility other than the one she was initially evaluated at. It was there that she was diagnosed with a stroke caused by neurological vasculitis, a serious and potentially life-threatening condition.

The high dose chemotherapy she was immediately started on was responsible for her hair loss—but, more importantly, probably for saving her life. The patient was rehabilitated at another step-down facility after hospital discharge and subsequently sent home.

Having gotten my name and contact information from a mutual acquaintance, she reached out to me in the hope that I could help her pick up the pieces, assisting her in making some sense out of a scenario I see played out far more often than I care to admit—but reality prevents me from denying.

The most I can offer her as pleading orbs meet mine from across the table is to say, in many ways, I've been there, too—and that I understand, firsthand, how it feels to be dismissed—and how unfair it is. Yet, even as the words spill from my lips, my ears hear them as far too inadequate an explanation for someone who was not only dismissed and demeaned, but lead to believe her condition was psychiatric rather than physical when, in reality, she required neuro surgery. What else could this woman have done to communicate how seriously ill she was to the physicians she placed her trust in? (Disconcertingly it is heartbreakingly true stories such as these that leaves me unsurprised to learn of the high percentage of misdiagnosis in our country.)

Sadly, the more this patient shares, through bulging, tear-brimmed eyes, the more I can't help but silently consider what a flawed system we have, to some extent, for this to happen. There is no way a patient can PROVE they have neuro-vasculitis, yet, without being able to do so, she was suspected, (and close to being admitted for!), of having a psychiatric illness. To say my heart cries for this severely ill patient, for all she has been through—and the uncompassionate treatment she was subjected to—is an understatement. To find adequate words to verbalize my disappointment in the medical professionals initially associated with evaluation of her case—IMPOSSIBLE!

***

I can't conclude this section without discussing the inarguable vulnerability even the most secure people feel, as a helplessness foreign to them replaces their independence, when they become hospital patients—and understandably so. Your clothes are taken away and replaced by some skimpy hospital gown, you are assigned a bed from which you may have to ask permission to get up and go to the bathroom, (if allowed to do so at all!), you are told when you can get washed up, brush your teeth, etc. Discharge dates are far more influenced by your doctor than you, sometimes causing a patient to ask himself why he agreed to the admission in the first place—particularly when no diagnosis and/or effective treatment resulted from it.

It is not hard to picture why patients in such controlling environments would find it difficult to confront physicians from whom they feel they are not getting answers—but they must. Doing so can save their lives or, at the very least, lead to accurate diagnoses. There comes a time when no matter how nice a person you are, you have to put your own health before that of your doctor's feelings. You have the right to multiple opinions—a right I strongly recommend exercising if you are not satisfied with—or question—the diagnosis you've received.

In addition, hospitals have patient advocates on staff for your benefit. Employ their assistance in addressing changes you require, including those you are reticent to initiate yourself. Usually their contact information is shared with you shortly after admission. If not, ask one of the nurses for it and leave it readily assessable at your bedside.

Keep in mind other, often less vulnerable resources at your disposal, including family and friends. If comfortable doing so, share with them any needs and/or doubts about the care you are receiving, the diagnosis you are being treated for, etc. (Be sure you give the medical staff permission, not only verbally but in writing, advising them of whom you want them to share your medical information with, if that is your choice.) It's your life—fight for it!

CHAPTER FIFTEEN

Exploring Solutions

"Success does not consist of never making mistakes, but in never making the same one a second time." —George Bernard Shaw

Inarguably, the ink on previous pages of this book spelled out words that described unacceptable numbers and cases of medical errors and/or misdiagnoses which could—and have in some situations—proven life-threatening.

Barely able to keep up with typing that almost involuntarily spits out verbiage on previously blank sheets of paper—no longer plain white but modified with black alphabetic characters that, when put together, form words—the seemingly automatic transformation leaves me somewhat in awe. Logically, it should not as I'm responsible for researching the numerous and encouraging steps currently being taken to decrease misdiagnoses errors—a cause I can't advocate for enough. In contrast to the negative statistical publicity reported over the past decade-plus, I can only surmise that my enthusiasm to share such positive information with the reader - about studies and safety checks that offer a significantly increased sense of security regarding medical care currently in place—caused my fingers to type as though they were on steroids. So without further delay, following are some of the recently developed modifications to improve patient safety and encourage accurate diagnoses:

* * *

According to The Wall Street Journal, (WSJ), "How Hospitals Are Preventing Misdiagnosis", (6:39 A.M., November 19, 2013), state of the art computer technology is now being utilized to reduce diagnostic mistakes. Reporter Laura Landro informs readers that cross-checking methods are currently employed to avoid errors and overlooked information, potentially resulting in dangerous and expensive misdiagnosis. Statistics like those reported by researchers at Johns Hopkins University reveal that missed diagnoses result in permanent damage or deaths in up to 160,000 patients per year. Considering that the frequency of occurrence in this specific category reflect a higher prevalence than other medical mistakes, the use of computer technology logic to avoid misdiagnosis is an encouraging step in an innovative direction. (Ironically, my husband, driven by his I.T. background and desperation to resolve my then-unidentified "medical mystery", recommended systems capable of executing detailed scrutiny, (of symptom-stumping afflictions), decades ago—unfortunately at a time when computer technology was still new to the general public—and, consequently too foreign for objective comprehension of its diagnostic potential by the specialist he proposed it to.) However, as a previously-misdiagnosed, rare disease patient I can't advocate enough that physicians utilize such technology for their "mystery diagnoses patients". Repeatedly stressing this, (though I'm not sure I can do it enough), I continue to contend that with the thousands of rare diseases in existence, it is unrealistic to expect physicians to memorize the symptoms of every one. To think that the infrequently seen, unexplained and potentially life-threatening afflictions of undiagnosed patients could be entered into a computer with the capability of, by quickly sorting through them, identifying each into specific categories associated with one of these rare diseases, while technologically cross-checking to further validate the diagnosis, is encouraging and hopeful, not only for future patients—but the medical profession as well.

One of the most innovative I.T. developments I've come across is known as "Isabel", named after the founders' daughter—who faced a dangerously close-to-fatal misdiagnosis. Troubled by how such a serious medical mistake could occur, her parents—Charlotte and Jason Maude—returned several weeks later to the hospital where their child's distressingly-inaccurate diagnosis occurred. Interrogating a staff member as to how this could happen, they were told, "clinical ignorance", followed by an explanation eluding to too little education and exposure by younger practitioners. Recognizing that if it happened to one, it could happen to others—and with a solution in mind—Isabel was "born". Comprised of a checklist of numerous symptoms, it offers a logical approach to determine if a mistakenly-labeled idiopathic syndrome is, in fact, a specific disease. Used with "mystery illnesses", in particular, I see this as a godsend in recognizing rare and/or atypical presentations at their earliest, most treatable stages. Impressively, this program has merited supportive publication in more than 30 medical articles. Its accuracy is corroborated by its 90% score on a survey conducted by a respected U.S. evaluation company for informational technology, (KLAS). Thanks to innovative parents who understood, firsthand, the desperation and danger misdiagnosed patients, (and their families), can encounter, a negative situation turned positive—in a way that is now helping reduce diagnostic errors all over the world.

***

As described by Heather Hellman, in "Patients Who Help Train Doctors", (October 10, 2000), Tulane University developed a comprehensive program to prepare medical students for what they will encounter when they graduate and establish practices of their own. Determined that they leave with the background needed to effectively do so, in addition to clinical skills such as executing examinations while demonstrating an understanding of what they should be looking for, active listening is a priority given equal attention. Students are taught not to interrupt patients when they are speaking and to hear what they say open-mindedly. To encourage and evaluate their success in doing so, standardized patients, (often hired to coach and emulate actual patients, with the skills to teach and score medical students assessing them), are utilized. They serve two functions: 1) providing instruction and detailed feedback as students conduct exams on them and 2) as actors, they present with specific, pre-arranged syndromes generated by the medical school. In the latter, the "patients" have been tutored in presenting their symptoms, how detailed the histories they give should be, etc.—providing enough information for the student to determine a diagnosis on his own, without giving it to him.

In my opinion, Tulane University—(and any others employing similar, professionally-coached, hands-on, immediate feedback training), is on the cutting edge of assuring innovative and comprehensive preparation of future physicians. What I found especially meaningful—based on a void I experienced, firsthand, with specialists in the past who did not reflect such open-minded awareness and sensitivity, is that in addition to ascertaining necessary clinical skills have been mastered, Tulane requires medical students to demonstrate to patients that what they say is as much a priority as what the doctor does. I have no doubt that promoting teamwork such as this, conducive to a non-condescending environment, enables optimal communication— resulting in earlier and more accurate diagnoses.

***

In "A System to Describe and Reduce Medical Errors in Primary Care, (Victoria Kaprielian, M.D., Trulsh Ostbye, M.D., PhD., Samuel Warburton, M.D., Devdutta Sangvai, M.D., MBA and Lloyd Michener, M.D.), I learned Duke University developed and implemented a program to report, analyze and address errors at the primary care level, where most care is provided. The goal is that if errors could be noticed at this initial stage, there would be reduced hospitalizations, costs and malpractice claims, resulting in optimal doctor/patient relationships.

***

Some of the Information I found most thought-provoking and informative was that shared by doctors who were, at some stage, patients themselves. The shoe-on-the-other-foot compassion their firsthand experiences generated changed how they treated their own patients—in a positive way—once they recovered and returned to their medical practices. While it is unfortunate that these physicians had to experience illnesses themselves—during this involuntary learning process—I think they should be commended for sharing the honest and eye-opening revelations they encountered as a result of their own medical challenges. It is through disclosure of firsthand observations such as these that improvements are initiated.

In "A Taste of My Own Medicine", Dr. Edward Rosenbaum was told there was nothing wrong with his vocal chords, (not true), and that his condition was psychological. "I really knew better. Too often doctors use that diagnosis to hide their failings," he stated. While he didn't argue the diagnosis, he did share how such an incorrect label could, under certain circumstances, obscure serious, even life-threatening errors. To read of a relative of his, who was given the same diagnosis only to die months later of a PHYSICAL illness, was heart-wrenching.

In one section he related how, though his words agreed with what his doctor said, his thoughts did not. He, like other patients, worried that challenging his physician's diagnosis would anger the professional in charge of his care, potentially resulting in inferior treatment. I, personally, am guilty of allowing intimidation, (in more than one instance—where I felt powerless), to override my own logic, resulting in my agreeing with a diagnosis and/or protocol which, though I didn't believe in, I didn't question, either. Having been hard on myself for my lack of assertiveness, in retrospect I was somewhat reassured when Dr. Rosenbaum shared through firsthand experience that not only patients—but physicians as well—demonstrate such vulnerabilities under challenging circumstances where their own health is involved. I respect him for the unpretentious and honest portrayal of medicine that he open-mindedly shared with lay people by going out on what might be considered a controversial limb, including professional information sometimes undisclosed. He demonstrated through example what we all know to be true—medicine is NOT an exact science. Mistakes can and will be made. How we react to and learn from those mistakes is OUR job. I, for one, learned a lot from this author!

* * *

In Lessons "From the Other Side": Teaching and Learning from Doctors' Illness and Narratives, author Jonathon Tomlinson discusses the accounts of several physician/patients. His objective in sharing their firsthand observations is to facilitate improvements. I think it was very selfless and educational of him and the other doctors to confide their eye-opening, personal experiences so that others can benefit. While intimate stories can be difficult to publicize, (tell me about it!), the positive ramifications from doing so far outweigh any initial reluctance involved. I hope the open-minded disclosure I've seen developing lately becomes a trend, not only by physicians but patients as well. I'm convinced that working together we can significantly lower misdiagnosis statistics.

***

Kate Granger, a terminally ill young doctor with metastatic sarcoma wrote a book, "The Other Side", based on her firsthand experience as a patient. Intending to introduce medical staff, unexposed personally, to what it is like to be in a hospital bed—rather than caring for someone who is—she unselfishly, (while challenged by severe illness and undoubtedly depleted energy), took the time to educate health professionals to a reality she lived: how powerfully medical staff interactions impact patients—and not always in a positive way. "If being ill has taught me anything about being a doctor", she shares, "it is the importance of seeing a patient as a person and not merely a condition or disease set in a hospital bed."

Due to a revelation she found distressingly unacceptable, (and understandably so!), during one of her hospitalizations—that care was administered to her by individuals who didn't even introduce themselves in advance—she founded the #hello my name is campaign. Determined to make a positive difference, her goal in doing so was to emphasize—beyond good manners—how desperately fragile patients, at such insecure, challenging and scary stages of health— need to feel "humanness" from their health care workers in order to trust them, (and she's right!). Unfortunately, the kind of perception it took for her to identify and recognize the need to make changes, to an objectionable situation I can far-more-personally-than-I'd-like relate to, often requires firsthand experience to fully comprehend.

It disheartens me to report that this dedicated young physician— who, despite limited time left, still shared what her firsthand dire circumstances taught her so that others could benefit—passed at the age of 34. In my opinion, in her short career as a doctor, through her determination and selfless way, she contributed more toward understanding what it feels like to be a patient—and how treatment can be improved—than many physicians who have been in practice for decades. Thank you, Kate!

***

From "When a Doctor Becomes a Patient", by Wendy Schlessel Harpham, M.D., F.A.C., (Ladies Home Journal, Nov. 2000), readers learn of her incurable form of non-Hodgkin's lymphoma. After bravely enduring multiple aggressive chemotherapy treatments which caused her to go in and out of remissions, it became disconcertingly clear to her that at the time she was unable to resume her internal medicine practice—a reality she extremely regretted. However, determined to continue to represent the nurturing profession she chose, she creatively found a way to continue to help others by combining her medical background with that of her firsthand disease experience. Instead of going to the office every day, which the fatigue associated with her illness made prohibitive, she engaged in educational activities over which she had more control of her time management, including public speaking and writing. To date she has authored several books and, by turning a negative situation into a positive one, is an asset to the medical community as they treat others with not only her disease—but those challenged with a variety of serious illnesses. It is inspiring people like her, who demonstrate how to keep fighting despite adversity—even when it means making unexpected career changes, whether temporary or permanent—that encourage others not to give up.

***

In "How to Improve Doctors' Bedside Manners" by Shefali Luthra, Kaiser Health News, Sunday September 13, 2015, Martha Hayward, leader in public and patient engagement efforts at the Institute for Healthcare Improvement, (MA.) asserts, "We don't train toward lifestyle understanding." In the same article that this concern was "voiced", it is noted that doctors' curriculums historically did not include sensitivity training. Demanding workloads and high stress were attributed to physicians being seen as "brusque, condescending or inconsiderate". According to a 2011 study, only slightly more than half of hospitalized patients acknowledged compassion in their health care experience—which is ironic given that doctors and patients BOTH agree on the importance of kindness. Encouragingly, however, these issues are positively being addressed as patient expectations are shared more assertively than in the past. By gradually influencing physicians to incorporate more active listening, patients are instrumental in promoting and receiving increased sensitivity to their needs—a fact corroborated in surveys that replace previous criticism generated by its lack, with comments reflecting greater satisfaction. Rather than the traditional training which emphasizes asking what the problem is and zeroing in exclusively on diagnosis, lifestyle understanding is now an integral consideration in preparing future physicians.

Medical facilities and doctors already in private practice are also concertedly making efforts to improve their bedside manners. Not only does doing so increase their patient load, given that patients are assuming an increasing amount of financial responsibility for their care and are more entitled than ever to demand input into who they see—but Medicare reimbursement to hospitals can be influenced by patient satisfaction surveys.

According to Tim Vogus, associate professor of Management at Vanderbilt University, his research—which explores the relationship between institutions that use techniques to assure physicians' responsiveness and compassion—(ex. Cleveland Clinic, the University of Michigan and various Catholic hospitals)—reveals a positive correlation between those that do, and better scores on patient satisfaction surveys.

Partners Healthcare, (MA.), and medical schools including Duke, are requiring students to enroll in classes stressing empathy development and implementation. Such instruction is also available to physicians already in practice.

In addition to medical information, it is recommended that personal facts be included in a patient's chart—which goes a long way in indicating how much your physician heard not only about your physical condition—but the degree he cares about your life style in general. For example, when you haven't seen a specialist in three months—during which he has undoubtedly seen hundreds of patients in between, who could potentially distract him from the details of your case—but he asks how your cruise was, you know he listened to what you previously talked about and cared enough to document it. A personal call, (regardless of how long or short in duration), does wonders to lift the spirits of a seriously ill patient touched by the fact that though the doctor may not have a cure—and is probably swamped with work—took the time to see how his patient was doing. Especially in cases of those challenged by a serious health crisis, it is the little things that really do make a difference—and hug a patient's heart when they need it most.

One of the positive techniques I was unaware of—but

impressed me most—was the way patient evaluations are utilized by the University of Rochester Medical Center. Not only do they monthly recognize physicians noted for their compassion, how well they hear and interpret what their patients report, whether they find a little extra time to stay with them and answer questions in patients' terms, etc.—they also address negative comments in a positive, non-demeaning way, through physician coaching. In such situations, those involved receive objective coaching from other doctors who observe them practicing and advise them as to how they translate the way they interact with patients. Following such exercises, there is discussion regarding how the patient-criticized physician could have demonstrated more compassion and, where indicated, role playing is incorporated. "Coaching changes doctors' behavior, according to Susan McDaniel, a psychologist in charge of Rochester's coaching program. They're exhibiting skills that they weren't exhibiting before".

When researching this article, I found I related to and agreed with much of what it reported based on my own firsthand experience—most particularly, the importance of medical staff introducing themselves when entering an exam room--and the positive correlation between how patients treated respectfully are more compliant with following a physician's prescribed regiment, while dismissive, condescending or rushed demeanors can result in just the opposite. Inarguably, a relaxed, trusting environment, where the patient is allowed to feel like a team member, is conducive to volunteering more pertinent medical information—again, ideally enabling an earlier and more accurate diagnosis.

***

In Need of Diagnosis(INOD)

In addition to new programs currently being instituted,

it is important to acknowledge those which have been in place for years—continuing to work toward eradicating or at least lessening statistics for misdiagnosis. One that comes to mind is In Need of Diagnosis, a patient support resource that was developed in 2006 through the dedication and compassion of an undiagnosed and since-passed patient, Marianne Gianetti. Due to her firsthand experience, she understood what it was like to be mislabeled as a hypochondriac and/or assumed that her illness was no more than a psychosomatic condition. Having had an appreciation for the unacceptable number of rare diseases that often went undiagnosed and/or misdiagnosed, through personal contact by phone and countless hours dedicated to her determination to help others, Marianne reached out and touched the lives and hearts of more seriously ill people than almost anyone I know—helping them in any way she could.

One of her biggest concerns was that there was no such thing as a doctor specializing in diagnosis. While all physicians utilize the skill, she wanted someone a patient could go to specifically when the physicians they'd seen had not been able to determine what was wrong—more like a mystery illness specialist. She also felt that by requiring doctors to select a diagnostic code there was too much pressure and guesswork involved and that there should be one for "diagnosis unknown", and I have to agree. With the number of rare disorders there are, rather than trying to fit a patient into a category just to give their symptoms a name, recognizing that the illness is not yet identified will avoid misdiagnosis and buy time to do further research into the real cause.

INOD receives so many calls per year for help from patients often ready to give up that it is a challenge just to keep up with them—but they do. Remarkably they manage to give personal thought to every patient's particular needs, providing information based on their specific situations. Where appropriate, they research resources closest to the patient's home and share them. They not only service nationally but internationally, as well. Marianne worked hard turning a negative health experience into a positive dream so that she could help others. Her legacy lives on for the rest of us to benefit as the organization continues to exist, with board members consisting not only of various medical professionals but members from multiple walks of life. I am proud to say Marianne invited me to serve on it—which proved to be a very educational and eye-opening period of my life, during which my compassion for undiagnosed and/or misdiagnosed patients intensified beyond words. Our world wouldn't understand the lyrics, "How Can People Be So Heartless"? if everyone answered this organization's phones for just one day—trust me, hearing the variety of rare physical challenges called in—that most of us can't even fathom exist—would transform heartlessness to compassion. May God bless you, Marianne, for your efforts in making that happen!

***

The Undiagnosed Disease Program

Recognizing the need to address patients with severe conditions for which they, and their physicians, had no names and/or effective treatment, The Undiagnosed Disease Program was "born" at the National Institutes of Health, (NIH), in 2008 in Bethesda, MD. Designed to incorporate the very best resources in multiple specialties, this in-demand program receives requests from physicians nationwide for help with their "mystery illness" patients. As one would expect, there are far less availabilities than patients seeking them. To qualify, personal physicians submit medical records and complete forms, as do the patients, themselves. If fortunate enough to be selected, a week-long evaluation at the facility ensues. Among others, specialties evaluating individual cases during this time could include: endocrinology, immunology, cardiology, genetics and more. Having contacted staff members, attended web meetings in association with it and talked to individuals applying for admission, I couldn't be more impressed with The Undiagnosed Disease Program. The fact that such a renowned institution recognized this need—and formally established a program addressing it—should be reassuring to all of us. This is some of the most encouraging news I've come across since pursuing a rare disease diagnosis. To say this program is an asset in preventing misdiagnosis would be an understatement. How fortunate we are to have it in place!

***

The Coalition to Improve Diagnosis

Inarguably, the multiple strides being taken to reduce misdiagnosis complement one another, with a united goal in mind. It is like one positive strategy after another is being introduced to remedy the unacceptable statistics that scare patients—and their families. A highly impressive representation of this includes the cohesive efforts of a collaborative plan to reduce misdiagnosis. Comprised of a variety of pertinent voices, The Coalition to Improve Diagnosis was established to address specific causes for statistically proven unacceptable medical misdiagnosis. According to Dr. Paul Epner, Medical Chairman of the Coalition and Vice President of the Society to Improve Diagnosis in Medicine, (SIDM), "Engaging leading health care organizations, professional societies and patients is an essential step in improving the quality of care patients receive and in reducing harm that can result from diagnoses that are inaccurate, missed, or inappropriately delayed". "Physicians excel at diagnosis, but errors or delays in reaching the right diagnosis still create harm and we can do better", states Mark L. Graber, MD, SIDM president and founder. "The vision of our society is to ensure that diagnosis is accurate, timely and efficient. The Coalition to Improve Diagnosis will be the catalyst for changes in practice needed to realize this vision."

With input and/or sanction from , among others, the following: American Board of Internal Medicine, American Association of Nurse Practitioners, American College of Emergency Physicians, American College of Physicians, National Patient Safety Foundation, Society to Improve Diagnosis in Medicine, Society for Health Risk Management, American Board of Medical Specialties, consumers, patients and educators, clearly a conglomerate of much-appreciated and long overdue expertise comprises this essential board. From medical professionals who objectively recognize and take responsibility for misdiagnosis due to errors in their field, to firsthand recipients of medical mistakes, I'm optimistic that this coalition and logical approach toward research and assessment of the causes leading to currently reported misdiagnosis statistics will significantly decrease them.

Toward this goal, the National Academies of Science, Engineering and Medicine generated a report reflecting their findings, along with a plan intended to address preventable errors and/or delays in diagnosis that their research uncovered. Following are the eight suggestions documented in this report:

1) Facilitate more effective teamwork in the diagnostic process among healthcare professionals, patients and families.
2) Enhance healthcare professional education and training in the diagnostic process.
3) Ensure that health IT supports patients and professionals in the diagnostic process.
4) Develop and employ approaches to identify, learn from, and reduce diagnostic errors and near-misses in clinical practice.

5) Establish a work system and culture that supports the diagnostic process and improvements in diagnostic performance.
6) Develop a reporting environment and medical liability system that facilitates improved diagnosis through learning from diagnostic errors and near-misses.
7) Design a payment and care delivery environment that supports the diagnostic process.
8) Provide dedicated funding for research on the diagnostic process and diagnostic errors.

(Information for this section was compiled from a variety of sources which include: "The Coalition to Improve Diagnosis" by Megan Wood, August 27, 2015, Health Management.org, New "Coalition to Address Diagnostic Errors", Hospital and Health Networks, September 22, 2015 by Marty Stempniak and "Improving Diagnosis in Healthcare", The National Academies of Sciences, Engineering and Medicine, Health and Medicine Division, September 22, 2015.)

* * *

Although unable to locate the source, I recall reading several years ago of a program that sounded like an excellent way to teach medical students firsthand compassion by intentionally exposing them to some of the challenges their patients, (particularly the elderly), incur. From what my own aging brain cells allow me to recall, the students were confronted with various complicated and difficult-to-function-with situations as "patients" themselves. Some had to smear petroleum jelly on their lenses to learn what life is like challenged by impossible-to-wipe-away smudged, blurry vision; others were given cotton to stuff in their ears to demonstrate firsthand understanding and appreciation of the hearing they had as opposed to what many of their patients did not; crutches were distributed to a few, while fingers of some were taped together— among other "disabilities" the students temporarily incurred, the goal of this impressive pre-med environment was to instill empathy for potential patients in their futures—by attempting to prepare them through replicating, firsthand, physical complications they could present with.

I can't imagine such impressive strides, toward replicating what they will encounter once in actual practice, not positively influencing medical students. Certainly, a patient who can't hear a physician, (and may be too embarrassed to admit it), is not going to answer his doctor's questions accurately, compromising the value of the history he provides. One who is sight-challenged may not be prescription-compliant because he is unable to read the instructions on the bottle, especially considering the miniscule print too often utilized in an effort to cram detailed directions on far-too-small labels. Awareness of these and other challenges can mean an earlier and accurate diagnosis—and I commend instructors who employ such creative and intentionally-difficult-to-forget ways to emphasize that reality. (I only wish I knew who developed this program so I could give them proper credit, as even searching the internet was unrevealing as far as locating the source.)

***

According to a report by Lesley Stahl on a 60 Minutes segment, produced by Shari Finkelstein, that aired on Sunday, November 27th, 2016, there is an area in a region of the Andes, (Antioquia, Columbia), with the greatest concentration in the world of people who carry a rare genetic mutation that makes them 100% sure to develop early-onset Alzheimer's. Presenting itself in their forties, unfortunately patients usually succumb to it within ten years. Because of the high propensity and atypically young age of patients generated from this concentrated area, the National Institute of Health is conducting research to try to determine why. Currently patients are being interviewed by neurologists who, thanks to well-preserved and detailed church records, are able to piece together histories of biological fathers and grandfathers having exhibited similar symptoms at young ages. (According to these older accounts, what we now call Alzheimer's was then labeled "softening of the brain".)

Interestingly, a Harvard professor's talk in Bogotá was the impetus for the in depth—and initially unplanned studies, now being conducted. At its conclusion, someone in the audience approached him to say he knew of a family in which several members had the disease—and that it went back many generations—to the 1800's.

Thanks to this professor's commitment to early and accurate diagnosis—and willingness to extend his stay to do further research—we are learning more about the genetic component, with emphasis focused on whether it is possible to detect the propensity for the disease before it manifests in a patient. While unlikely in the past, the community currently being studied may be the exception. Based on a gene mutation in 50% of family members, P.E.T. scans are being conducted on those who have the gene but are asymptomatic to date. What has been revealed is that amyloid plaques can be seen in their brains more than ten years before the disease manifests with noticeable symptoms.

Currently, they are scientifically exploring ways to remove plaques from the brains of such individuals, the goal being to learn if doing so will eliminate the severity of the disease when it does materialize.

* * *

In concluding this section, suffice it to say that as a patient I found this small representation of the many efforts the medical community is continually making to explore reasons for—and consequently eliminate incidents of misdiagnosis—most reassuring.

CHAPTER SIXTEEN

Hopeful Horizons and Firsthand Reflections

"When the whole world is silent, even one voice becomes powerful."

—Malala Yousafzai

"I alone cannot change the world, but I can cast a stone across the water to create many ripples." —Mother Teresa

Inarguably, in my mind the prognosis for misdiagnosis is dependent on a variety of circumstances—probably first and foremost, the severity of the inaccurately diagnosed disease, followed by how long it takes to be identified correctly and, as a result, appropriately treated. Even at that, the possibility exists that it is recognized too late or, despite the medical community's most vigilant and best-intentioned intervention, is incurable.

From what I've encountered, however, the more open-minded the physicians, the more optimistic my prognoses have been. I believe it is the tenacious doctors who continue to search for answers, in some cases despite normal test results, (keeping in mind that medicine is not an exact science), who eventually solve medical mysteries that have challenged their colleagues beyond answers. Because of this, I don't regret one minute of the time I dedicated to researching what I consider "the best of the best" specialists, as I am convinced becoming their patient has had life- saving consequences. Being an undiagnosed and/or misdiagnosed patient, I deserve nothing less—nor do you!

* * *

Tears of the misdiagnosed are shed by some of the strongest people you will ever meet. Motivated by desperation to save lives that they are often the only ones aware are in jeopardy, patients with debilitating, severe, to-date idiopathic conditions struggle through horrific scenarios.

Inarguably, dealing with frequently life-threatening, rare diseases would be challenging in itself yet, disconcertingly many are forced to waste already compromised energy convincing skeptical physicians, relatives and friends that they are really ill. Cringing down deep inside whenever they hear how good they look, their reality is that they are time bombs ticking—with deafening warnings that, infuriatingly, despite their repeated screams for help appear ignored—especially by those they are convinced are capable of helping them most.

For decades, I lived in a world of unspeakable frustration, excruciating pain and indescribable fear—unable to convey the magnitude of my living hell—or, more importantly, to get help. Too much time elapsed before my diagnosis was confirmed—resulting in irreversible damage to major organs, most particularly my eyes. It scares and infuriates me beyond words to hear from a glaucoma specialist that had I been referred earlier, when I first sought help, my prognosis would have been much more optimistic. Instead, the goal is to try to prolong my vision for another decade.

* * *

Like snow that melts, trickling down roadside rocks in the Springtime, tears imbed trails down my cheeks, leaving their sticky residue for all the world to see—and truthfully, I don't care. Unlike the ones that have fallen in the past, these are relieved droplets. For more than twenty years, I've contended that misdiagnosis is one of the most serious mistakes the medical profession can make, (undoubtedly because of my firsthand "medical mystery" that remained unidentified for decades). In an effort to prevent others from enduring similar experiences, I advocate for patients who are desperately ill, with conditions for which they have no diagnosis. I've met people indescribably sick, only to be told when an accurate label could not be discovered, that it must be "psychological"—and my heart dripped with unseen compassionate tears for them, until they, too, went to specialists who unraveled their medical mysteries and treated their diseases appropriately.

Despite the fact that in many cases it may have taken years, (and in some, decades), before these patients received the long overdue answers and affirmations they deserved, I'm relieved they finally did. I, for one, credit this to the fact that there is now more transparency in misdiagnosis awareness, (a reality openly acknowledged in articles authored by various physicians, as well). With increased admission of professional mistakes to peers and/or patients, I see a trend in which medical care is changing—in a most positive way. Additionally, there is much to be learned from doctors who have been patients, themselves, when they share their observations and criticisms—the goal being that the same mistakes are not repeated.

Yet, regardless of the optimism these realizations evoke, I feel like a tourist not ready to leave vacation and depart for home. Convinced there is far more to discover but little time left, I'm not ready to end this book—but will I ever be? Rather than attribute my hesitation to "so little time left", I choose to believe my most recent—to-date daily—irreconcilable anaphylaxis constitutes yet another medical mystery, whose solution has yet to be identified, (if ever!). On the other hand, I'm encouraged regarding the many positive efforts I've discovered during my research for this book— introduced by the medical community—to decrease medical errors and associated misdiagnoses.

With my biological clock ticking seemingly faster with every decade, I'm at a loss to explain how reaching the age to qualify for a driver's license seemed to take forever, yet in the blink of an eye I'm approaching seventy, (almost). If I didn't know better, I'd swear there were less days in each successive year as we age through adulthood—or at least it seems so! While my guess is that readers are smiling as they identify firsthand with this phenomenon, my prayers are that they don't identify with unresolved medical mysteries. For me, personally, in regard to these unresolved, life-threatening anaphylactic symptoms, I end this portion of my medical journey on a hopeful note—that an answer is imminent— and a prayer that any undiagnosed patients reading this book get theirs as well.

At this point I want to publicize my sincerest thanks to the remarkably competent physicians I currently see. In truth, I wasn't always so fortunate. It took perseverance and assertiveness to assemble what I consider to be the very best team of specialists I could ask for—not to mention long distance travel to renown experts, pursuit of multiple opinions and the perception to recognize when it was time to say good-bye to doctors I felt were ineffective and/or dismissive.

Did you ever have a dream that was so good you didn't want to wake up? As though by clinging to every moment of it, you will it to continue—while extracting every positive message it allows you to take. That is how I feel under the care of my current doctors—almost as though part of their sincere concern can't be real—like in the snap of fingers I can wake up to the dismissal and lack of compassion I knew before. But unlike then, even during my darkest, scariest and most painful moments, these physicians don't tell me to find another doctor or to stop wasting their time when I am perfectly healthy—time that patients who are genuinely ill need—and deserve.

Inarguably, one of the most positive differences this time, as opposed to in the past, is the unmistakable "team" feeling I now know. I am truly as much a player in medical decisions as any of my doctors—a refreshing change I welcome. From the depth of our discussions there is no doubt that they respect my intelligence as much as I do theirs'. They listen attentively to observations I report and often act upon my suggestions. When they don't, they provide logical explanations as to why they won't work. I'm given the sincere impression that no question is ignorant and I'm never dismissed and/or rushed—and it feels good.

As I "think" these words an analogous image from childhood resurrects in my memory banks which, for this aging patient, is easier to retrieve than episodes that require short-term recollection. Like grains of sand filtering through a plastic sifter as I sit shaking it on the breezy ocean side, somehow tolerant of the stinging as the wind whips my gritty, salty hair onto my cheeks—(probably too preoccupied with the fun I'm having to let it stop me)—only the biggest and best pebbles don't fall through. That is how I think of the doctors I now see—those who exude the greatest amount of compassion and the most competent care I've ever received—not always easy to find but well worth the search.

Whatever you do, don't give up on the search—most importantly, remain true to yourself throughout the process. No one knows your body like you. If you think something is wrong, keep looking. Select those "pebbles" that stand out among the grains of sand. While it feels like I have enough grains from my search chasing answers to mystery diagnoses to build a whole city of sandcastles, I respect far more the limited but exceptional ones that stand out, too large to pass through my "adult sifter" to construct more than a toothpick-sized structure—and so will you!

May God bless all undiagnosed and/or misdiagnosed patients with the foresight to know where to turn for answers—and their medical professionals with the wisdom to recognize how to help.

MAKING A DIFFERENCE—ONE LIFE AT A TIME

A little boy walked carefully

Along a crowded beach,

Where starfish by the hundreds

lay there within his reach,

They washed up with each wave,

far as the eye could see,

and each would surely die,

If they were not set free,

So one by one he rescued them,

then heard a stranger call,

Surely it won't make a difference,

You can't save them all.

Tossing another back

in the direction of the warm sun

with deep compassion he said,

I made a difference to that one.

Adapted from "The Starfish

Thrower" by Loren Eiseley

About the Author

Eileen Radziunas has been exposed to the medical community both as a professional and a patient. Prior to diagnosis of her first autoimmune disease, she worked at a physicians' office and, subsequent to that, for a physical therapy practice. She attributes the medical knowledge she acquired, however, to her long diagnostic search necessitated by a rare illness, which involved cross-country travel for consultations with in excess of one hundred physicians representing multiple specialties. Advocating for the misdiagnosed and creating awareness of rare diseases through her other two books, "Lupus: My Search for a Diagnosis" and "But Doctor, You're Wrong!", she addressed medical students at both UCONN and YALE, was interviewed by radio stations and local newspapers and invited as the featured speaker at numerous book author luncheons, library signings and charitable events. Her first book was selected for inclusion in the World Trade Center Book Show at the Javitt's Center in N.Y.C. Through submission of sample chapters from her second book, she was awarded a Wesleyan University Writers' Conference Scholarship. On the local level, she established a support group for the chronically ill and successfully campaigned for Rare Disease Awareness Day in her town. Her primary reason for sharing such a personal story is to educate others so that no one else will have a story like hers to tell.

Made in United States
Troutdale, OR
11/03/2026

56847555R00133